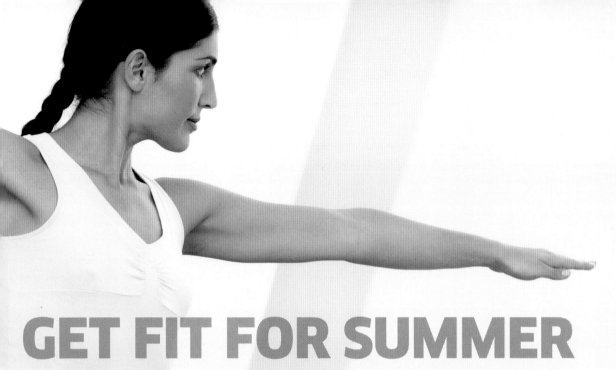

GET FIT FOR SUMMER
STRETCHING

Consultant
Joan Pagano

DK

London, New York, Melbourne, Munich, Delhi

Consultant Joan Pagano
Compiler and Editor Hilary Mandleberg
Editor Elizabeth Yeates, Neha Samuel
Designer Alison Shackleton, Neha Wahi
Stills Photography Ruth Jenkinson
Special Sales Creative Project Manager Alison Donovan
Pre-Production Producer Sarah Isle
Pre-Production Manager Sunil Sharma
Producer Charlotte Oliver
DTP Designers Rajdeep Singh, Satish Chandra Gaur

First published in Great Britain in 2014
by Dorling Kindersley Limited
80 Strand, London WC2R 0RL

Material in this publication was previously published in:
Stretching Workout (2010), Better Back Workout (2008), Abs Workout (2009),
Gentle Yoga (2008), Total Body Workout (2008), Everyday Pilates (2008)

A Penguin Random House Company

2 4 6 8 10 9 7 5 3 1
001-262103-Jan/2014

Health warning: All participants in fitness activities must
assume the responsibility for their own actions and safety.
If you have any health problems or medical conditions,
consult with your doctor before undertaking any of the
activities set out in this book. The information contained
in this book cannot replace sound judgement and good
decision making, which can help reduce risk of injury.

This edition produced for the Book People Ltd,
Hall Wood Avenue, Haydock, St Helens, WA11 9UL

Printed and bound in China by
South China Printing Co. Ltd.

Discover more at **www.dk.com**

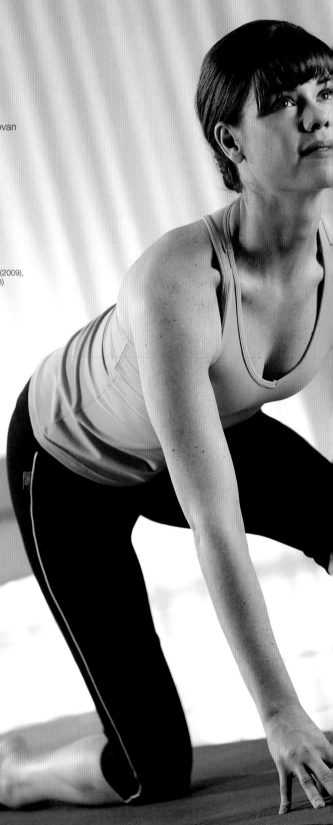

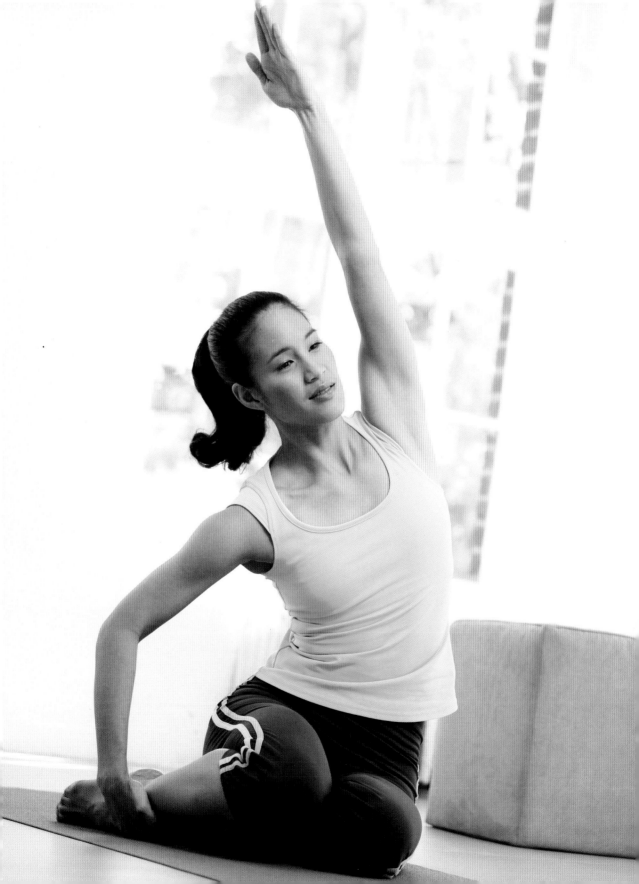

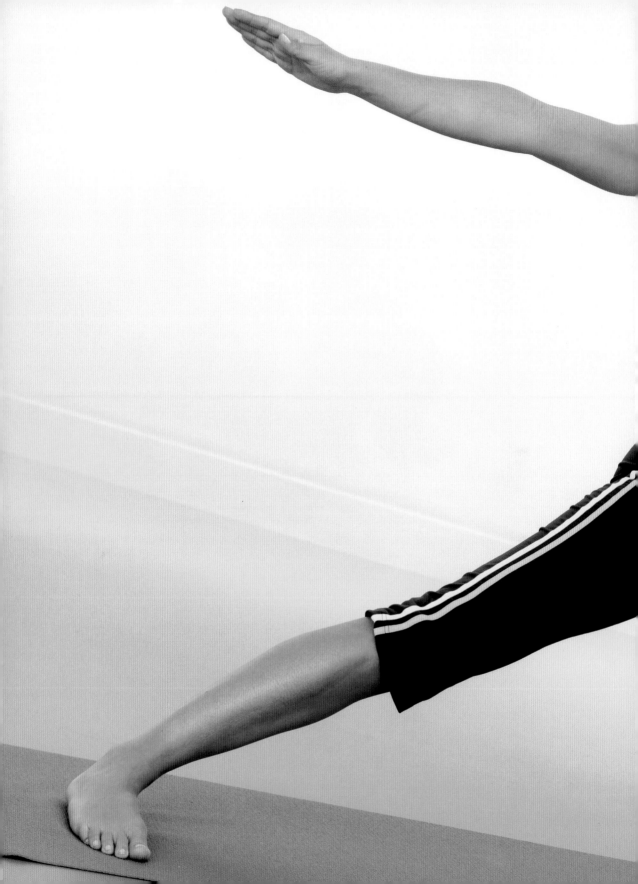

contents

before you begin   6

test your fitness   8

modify as needed   10

arm swing   12

arm circles   13

shoulder circles   14

elbow circles   15

butterfly stretch   16

back stretch   17

hanging stretch   18

shoulder ovals   19

baby rocks   20

knee pumps   21

ear tilt/chin tilt   22

overhead squeeze   23

side bends   24

cat and camel   25

front body opener   26

sidelying waist stretch   27

side stretch/spiral ab twist   28

cross-legged pose/twist   29

kneeling twist/thread the needle   30

balance point stretch   31

spine twist   32

the saw   33

'C' exercise   34

baby rolls   35

arm fans   36

fish stretch   37

modified cobra   38

cobbler stretch   39

inverse frog   40

quad stretch   41

thigh stretch   42

lying hamstring stretch   43

figure 4 stretch   44

kneeling cat   45

child's pose/downward dog   46

forward bend/mountain pose   47

pull-the-thread lunge   48

flat-back squat   49

the horse/triangle   50

warrior 2/side-angle stretch   51

oppositional lifts   52

advancing frogs   53

lunge opener   54

wide squat twist   55

fouetté stretch   56

the split   57

pigeon arabesque   58

angel flight stretch   59

calf stretch/spinal curve   60

spinal arch/child's pose   61

index   62

acknowledgments/about the authors   64

Before you begin

Stretching helps you stand taller, look younger and slimmer, and move more gracefully. Just a few minutes of stretching each day can help you stay flexible for a lifetime. And that's not all: Improving flexibility means better balance, less pain and fatigue, and even a clearer mind.

Flexibility training includes limbering exercises, lengthening stretches, and strengthening poses. This programme offers all three types by featuring a unique combination of techniques from fitness training, Pilates, yoga and physical therapy. You benefit from 'cross training,' a training routine involving several different forms of exercise that enhance overall health benefits, challenge you in new ways, and stimulate improvement.

You begin with Limbering (pp12–19), composed of exercises that loosen up your joints and release synovial (lubricating) fluid to make them work smoothly. These are movements that you repeat several or more times, to enhance the range of motion around the major joints of your upper body and spine. As you progress through the programme, you'll continue to find limbering exercises for your torso and lower body.

Lengthening stretches are positions that you hold for several breathing cycles while you coax the muscle into lengthening. When doing the Cross-legged pose and Twist (p29), for example, slowly stretch until you feel 'gentle pulling' in the target muscles, without any pain. Hold the position and then, as the muscle

relaxes, use your breath to advance a little deeper into the stretch. To avoid injury, move gradually without bouncing or jerking.

Strengthening poses, like those found in yoga and Pilates, require you to stabilize with certain muscles to hold the pose while you are performing additional movements. You may need to gather your core body strength, as in the Balance point stretch (p31) or Thigh stretch (p42). Some of the more advanced yoga positions (pp50–51) require strength and stability in the lower body while you move your torso and upper body. These are wonderful exercises that challenge your flexibility, strength, stability, balance, and coordination!

After you limber up, select 8 to 10 stretches from the programme for your routine. The colour-coding throughout the book indicates the level of difficulty of each exercise. You can progress through the levels of difficulty or mix and match.

If you only have a few minutes in the morning, just do the Limbering exercises (pp12–19). This is a perfect way to wake your body up and prepare it for the demands of the day. Before bedtime, pick some of the gentle stretches to counteract the wear and tear of the day.

Your ability to stretch is individual and depends on genetics as well as your daily habits. The unique structure of bones and the length of the soft tissue (muscles, tendons, and ligaments) surrounding them determine the joints' range of movement. Some joints, like those affected by arthritis, may be 'stiff' or restricted; others like those of a contortionist, 'loose' or hyper-mobile. You may also find that you are more flexible on one side than the other. Work within your genetic framework and make a habit of stretching, and there is no doubt that you will be able to enhance your flexibility.

Nothing makes you look older than poor posture and short, jerky movements. The constant downward pull of gravity and gradual dehydration of the body's tissues cause us literally to shrink over time, but stretching can help maintain height by lengthening the muscles around the spine and improving the mobility of the upper back. No beauty product will take years off your age as efficiently as just standing up a little straighter.

Muscles maintain the alignment of the skeleton in all positions. There is a natural tendency for some muscles to be short and tight, with others prone to being long andweak. Stretching can help offset this imbalance and improve alignment. Poor posture and alignment can cause pain: the muscles become chronically tired and strained, and more prone to injury. Headache, neck and shoulder tension, sciatica, and hip and knee pain can all be symptoms of this. In addition, shortened muscles are more at risk for injury. By enhancing your mobility, however, stretching increases your efficiency in all activities so that they require less effort and leave you feeling less tired.

Stretching also energizes you by releasing tension from the muscles and refreshing the mind. As anyone who has practised yoga knows, holding a stretch position is a type of moving meditation that reduces stress and promotes relaxation.

Safety notes: Have fun with these stretches! Stretching is not a competitive sport. Go at your own pace and avoid any positions that cause pain or discomfort. Move into the positions gradually, focus on the muscles you are targeting, and pay attention to stabilizing the rest of the body. Take your time and remember to breathe. Some people find stretching stressful (usually they have tight muscles) – breathing helps you relax into the stretch as well as advance deeper into, and get more out of, the position.

Joan Pagano

>> **test** your fitness

Before you start your training programme, you must check that it is safe for you to begin. Take the PAR-Q questionnaire on the opposite page, and if you are in any doubt about the state of your health, please see your doctor before becoming more physically active. The three tests below will help you to assess your fitness.

Track your progress

One way to measure muscular fitness is to count how many repetitions you can perform, or how many seconds you can hold a contraction. To see how you measure up, do the three exercises shown, which will assess your muscular endurance in the lower, middle, and upper body. Record your results, noting the date, and after three months of training, repeat the tests. When you reassess yourself, perform the same version of the exercise.

If you are just beginning to exercise, or coming back to it after a long break, you may prefer to perform your first assessment after two or three months of exercising on a regular basis. Before attempting the exercises, warm up first by moving your arms and legs briskly for five minutes.

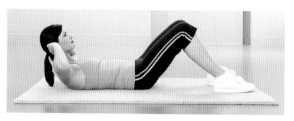

Middle body *Crunch with scoop*
Count how many crunches you can do consecutively without resting. This is not a full sit-up. Lift your head and shoulders no higher than 30° off the mat.

Your score

Excellent	50 reps or more
Good	35–49 reps
Fair	20–34 reps
Poor	20 reps or less

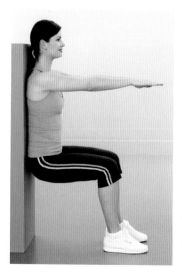

Lower body

Wall squat
Slide down until your thighs are parallel to the floor and hold the position for as long as you can. (If you cannot slide all the way down, go as far as you can.)

Your score

Excellent	
90 seconds or more	
Good	
60 seconds	
Fair	
30 seconds	
Poor	
less than 30 seconds	

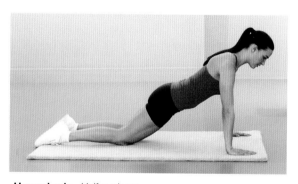

Upper body *Half push-up*
Inhale as you bend your elbows, lowering your chest to the floor. Exhale as you push up to the starting position. Count how many you can do consecutively without a rest.

Your score

Excellent	20 reps or more
Good	15–19 reps
Fair	10–14 reps
Poor	10 reps or less

PAR-Q AND YOU   A questionnaire for people aged 15 to 69 Physical Activity Readiness Questionnaire – PAR-Q (revised 2002)

Regular physical activity is fun and healthy, and increasingly more people are starting to become more active every day. Being more active is perfectly safe for most people. However, some people should check with their doctor before they start becoming much more physically active.

If you are planning to become much more physically active than you are now, start by answering the seven questions in the box below. If you are between the ages of 15 and 69, the PAR-Q will tell you if you should check with your doctor before you start. If you are over 69 years of age, and you are not used to being very active, check with your doctor.

Common sense is your best guide when you answer these questions. Please read the questions carefully and answer each one honestly: check YES or NO.

YES NO

1 Has your doctor ever said that you have a heart condition <u>and</u> that you should only do physical activity recommended by a doctor?

2 Do you feel pain in your chest when you do physical activity?

3 In the past month, have you had chest pain when you were not doing physical activity?

4 Do you lose your balance because of dizziness or do you ever lose consciousness?

YES NO

5 Do you have a bone or joint problem (for example, back, knee, or hip) that could be made worse by a change in your physical activity?

6 Is your doctor currently prescribing drugs (for example, water pills) for your blood pressure or heart condition?

7 Do you know of <u>any other reason</u> why you should not do physical activity?

If you answered YES to one or more questions

Talk with your doctor by phone or in person BEFORE you start becoming much more physically active or BEFORE you have a fitness appraisal.
Tell your doctor about the PAR-Q and which questions you answered YES.
• You may be able to do any activity you want – as long as you start slowly and build up gradually. Or, you may need to restrict your activities to those which are safe for you. Talk with your doctor about the kinds of activities you wish to participate in and follow his/her advice.
• Find out which community programmes are safe and helpful for you.

If you answered NO to all questions

If you answered NO honestly to all PAR-Q questions, you can be reasonably sure that you can:
• start becoming much more physically active – begin slowly and build up gradually. This is the safest and easiest way to go.
• take part in a fitness appraisal – this is an excellent way to determine your basic fitness so that you can plan the best way for you to exercise and live actively. It is also highly recommended that you have your blood pressure evaluated. If your reading is over 144/94, talk with your doctor before you start becoming much more physically active.

DELAY BECOMING MUCH MORE ACTIVE:
• if you are not feeling well because of a temporary illness such as a cold or a fever – wait until you feel better; or
• if you are or may be pregnant – talk to your doctor before you start becoming more active.

PLEASE NOTE:
If your health changes so that you then answer YES to any of the above questions, tell your fitness or health professional. Ask whether you should change your physical activity plan.

>> **modify** as needed

It's not a failing to change an exercise to suit your needs, whether it's because of pain, age, or stiffness. There's a back door to every stretch. Nor is it cheating to use props and modifications. It's just plain wise.

The body can move in multiple directions with a great deal of ease, yet people are often deterred from doing stretching exercises because they worry about feeling discouraged. We would all love to look like the models featured in this book, but use them to help you see the stretching exercises clearly, not to compare yourself with them.

Some of the stretches may feel a little strange or unusual, especially if you are new to exercise. Part of the reason we stretch in unusual positions is to identify our weak links, so pay attention and focus on what feels too tight, too loose, or painful.

If an exercise doesn't feel right, there's always a way to make it more accessible. Some people have trouble sitting on the floor because they have tight hamstrings, glutes, or tightness in the low back, or a combination of one or more of these. Sitting on a footstool, ottoman, towel, or bolster can give just the lift needed to make the stretch possible.

Knees should never hurt during stretching. If they feel painful, support them on pillows or bolsters to take the pressure off. If you are doing poses like this, another tip is to move the feet further from the groin.

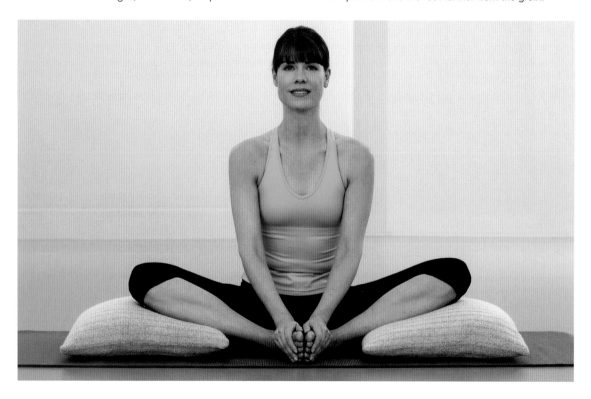

Pay special attention to your knees and monitor them for signs of pain or discomfort. 'No pain, no gain' definitely does not apply to these complex joints. If you need to, prop them up with pillows when you are sitting to take the strain off the ligaments. If they feel tender when you kneel on them in weight-bearing positions, support them with some form of padding. Straighten them out of a bent-leg position if it's uncomfortable. If one of the knees refuses to straighten, as it might in the Lying hamstring stretch (see p43), use a towel, belt, or strap to reach the foot.

You can increase or decrease the intensity of a stretch as it suits you (perhaps your body feels different on different days or at different times of day) by pulling or extending more or less. Breathing and relaxing help you stretch further. Alternatively, try modulating the intensity of a stretch by elongating in a progression from one to ten, and then reducing it. The level of intensity should never go into the 'strain zone' and you should not have extreme pain after you have performed your stretches. Remember: compare only yourself to yourself to make the greatest gain.

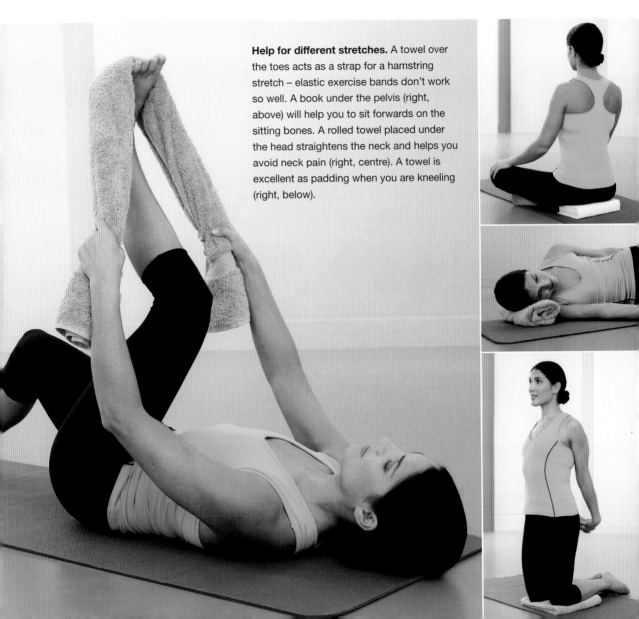

Help for different stretches. A towel over the toes acts as a strap for a hamstring stretch – elastic exercise bands don't work so well. A book under the pelvis (right, above) will help you to sit forwards on the sitting bones. A rolled towel placed under the head straightens the neck and helps you avoid neck pain (right, centre). A towel is excellent as padding when you are kneeling (right, below).

>> arm swing

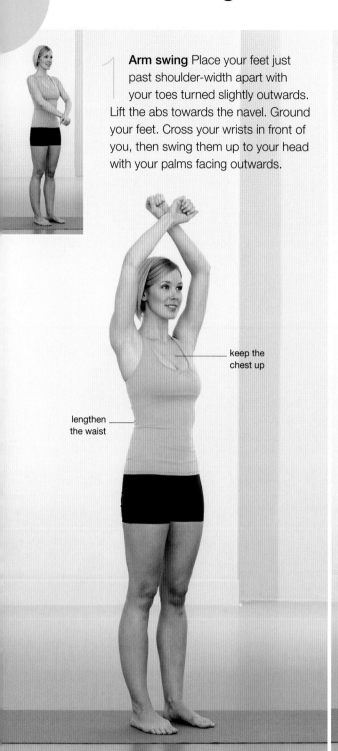

1 **Arm swing** Place your feet just past shoulder-width apart with your toes turned slightly outwards. Lift the abs towards the navel. Ground your feet. Cross your wrists in front of you, then swing them up to your head with your palms facing outwards.

2 Swing your hands back and behind your hips so they touch together. Rhythmically swing your arms up and back using this motion 7 more times.

keep the chest up

lengthen the waist

swing the hands back

>> arm circles

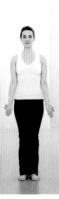

3 **Arm circles** With your heels together, work your glutes and hamstrings to rotate your feet slightly outwards. Shift your weight slightly forwards, arms by your thighs, palms facing forwards. Inhale, then exhale and raise your arms.

4 Flip the palms outwards and circle the arms down, exerting pressure as though the air were thick. Repeat 2 more times, then reverse the breath, inhaling on the raise and exhaling on the lower, for another 3 repetitions.

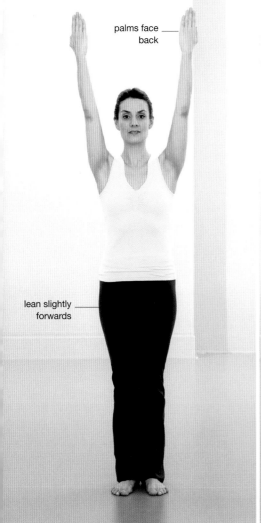

palms face back

lean slightly forwards

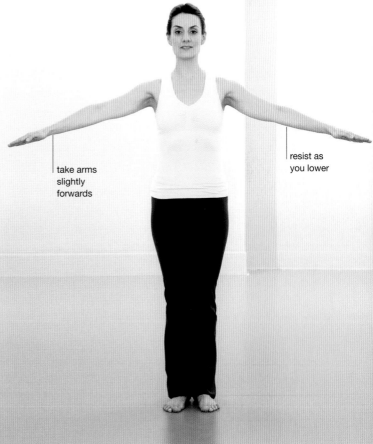

take arms slightly forwards

resist as you lower

>> shoulder circles

5 **Shoulder circles** With your legs shoulder-width apart, reach both arms overhead and clasp your fingers. Lengthen your tailbone towards the ground. Circle your arms, imagining making 4 circles on the ceiling with your hands. Return to centre.

6 Again, lift up and out of the waist and tighten the waist. Lengthen the tailbone. Reverse the movement with the hands, imagining making 4 more circles on the ceiling. Bring the arms down.

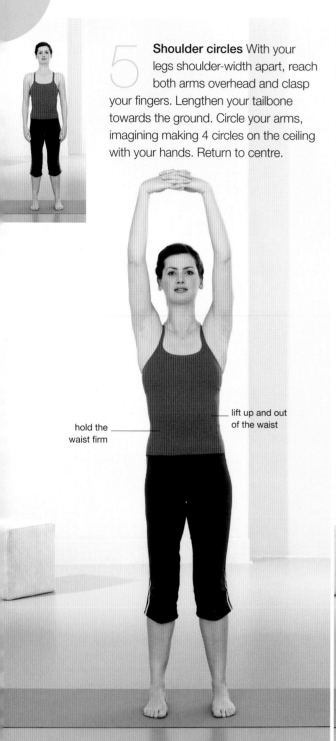

hold the waist firm

lift up and out of the waist

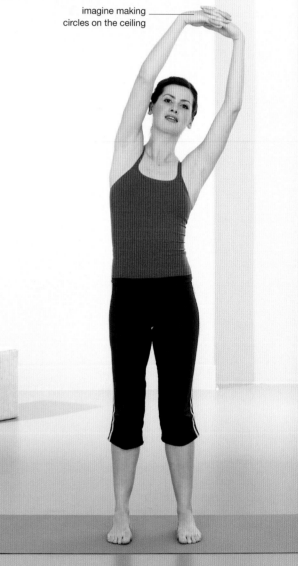

imagine making circles on the ceiling

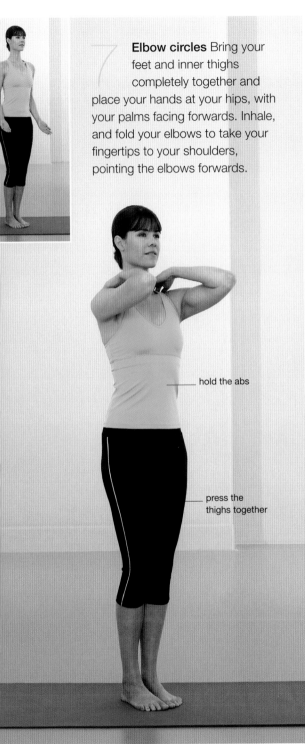

7 **Elbow circles** Bring your feet and inner thighs completely together and place your hands at your hips, with your palms facing forwards. Inhale, and fold your elbows to take your fingertips to your shoulders, pointing the elbows forwards.

hold the abs

press the thighs together

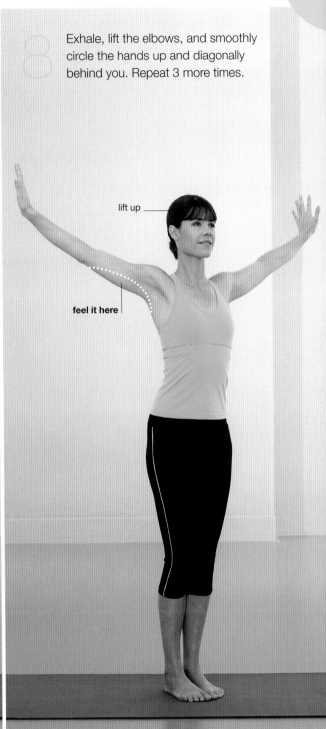

8 Exhale, lift the elbows, and smoothly circle the hands up and diagonally behind you. Repeat 3 more times.

lift up

feel it here

>> butterfly stretch

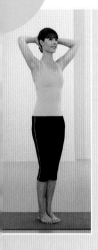

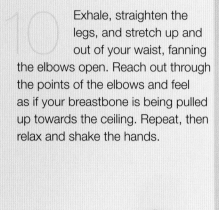

9 **Butterfly stretch** Stand with legs completely together and pressing the base of the big and little toes, and the middle of the heel of both feet on the floor. Lift your pelvic floor and pull your navel to your spine. Clasp your hands behind your head, inhale, and lift up and forwards from your waist. Simultaneously bow your head, bend your knee, and bring the elbows towards each other.

10 Exhale, straighten the legs, and stretch up and out of your waist, fanning the elbows open. Reach out through the points of the elbows and feel as if your breastbone is being pulled up towards the ceiling. Repeat, then relax and shake the hands.

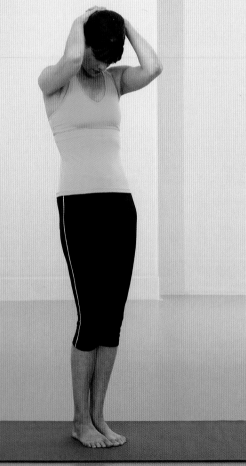

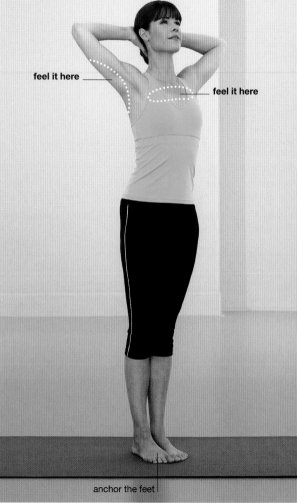

feel it here

feel it here

anchor the feet

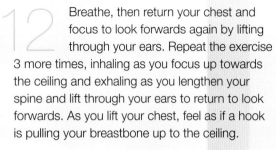

11 **Back stretch** Stand tall with your feet just less than hip-width apart. Align your head over your pelvis and pull your navel to your spine. Make fists with your hands and place your knuckles on your lower back. Exhale a little, then inhale as you lift your chest diagonally towards the ceiling.

12 Breathe, then return your chest and focus to look forwards again by lifting through your ears. Repeat the exercise 3 more times, inhaling as you focus up towards the ceiling and exhaling as you lengthen your spine and lift through your ears to return to look forwards. As you lift your chest, feel as if a hook is pulling your breastbone up to the ceiling.

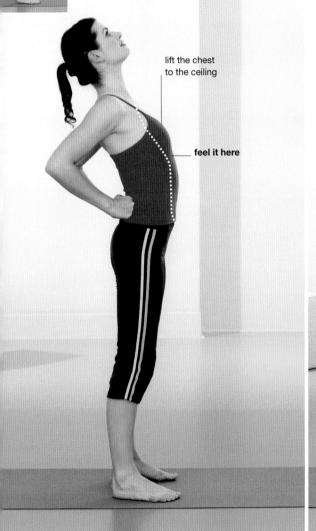

lift the chest to the ceiling

feel it here

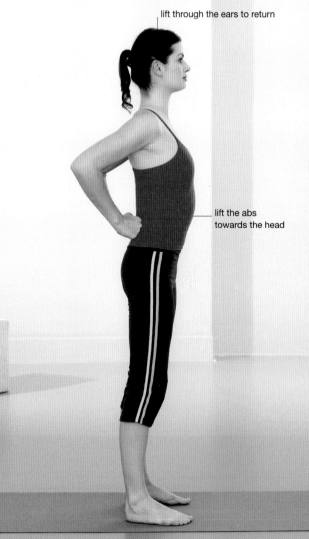

lift through the ears to return

lift the abs towards the head

>> hanging stretch

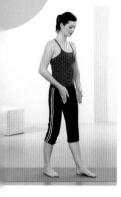

13 **Hanging stretch**
Stand with the legs about 3in (7.5cm) apart. Place the left foot ahead of the right with about a foot's-width between the legs. The toes point forwards. Cross the arms, hold the elbows and pull the navel firmly into the spine. Reach the elbows downwards.

14 Continue to reach the elbows down towards the floor. Stay in this rounded position, firmly holding the abs as you take 3 breaths. Carefully roll up, feeling as if your abs are walking up the front of your body. Repeat with the right food ahead of the left. Come back up and then relax.

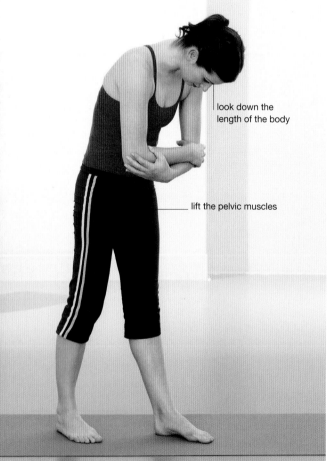

look down the length of the body

lift the pelvic muscles

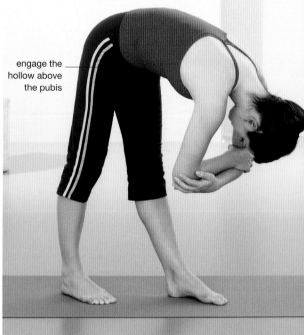

engage the hollow above the pubis

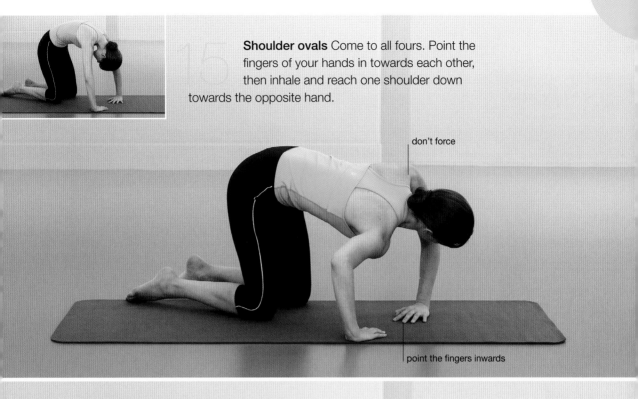

Shoulder ovals Come to all fours. Point the fingers of your hands in towards each other, then inhale and reach one shoulder down towards the opposite hand.

don't force

point the fingers inwards

Sweep the chest across the floor, past centre towards the other hand, then exhale and continue circling in the same direction as you round your back. Your shoulders should be making an oval in space. Keep going in the same direction for 2 more ovals, then change direction and reverse for 2 more ovals.

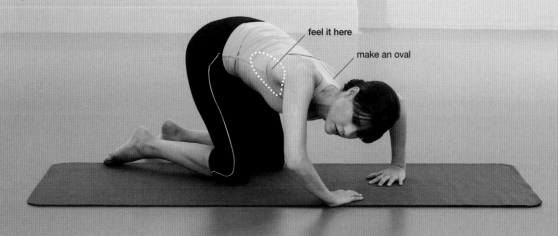

feel it here

make an oval

>> baby rocks

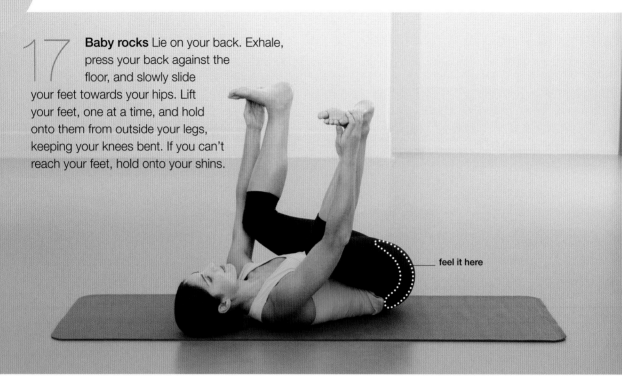

17 **Baby rocks** Lie on your back. Exhale, press your back against the floor, and slowly slide your feet towards your hips. Lift your feet, one at a time, and hold onto them from outside your legs, keeping your knees bent. If you can't reach your feet, hold onto your shins.

feel it here

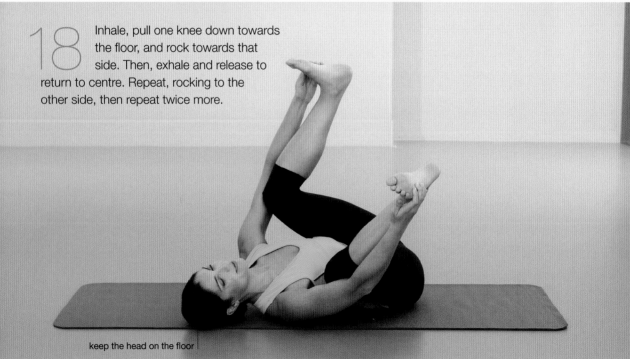

18 Inhale, pull one knee down towards the floor, and rock towards that side. Then, exhale and release to return to centre. Repeat, rocking to the other side, then repeat twice more.

keep the head on the floor

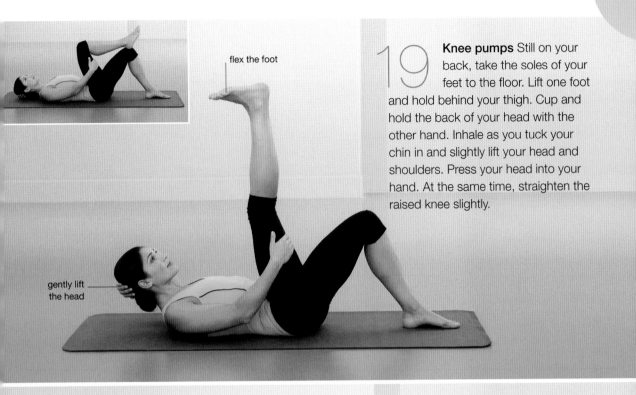

flex the foot

gently lift
the head

19 **Knee pumps** Still on your back, take the soles of your feet to the floor. Lift one foot and hold behind your thigh. Cup and hold the back of your head with the other hand. Inhale as you tuck your chin in and slightly lift your head and shoulders. Press your head into your hand. At the same time, straighten the raised knee slightly.

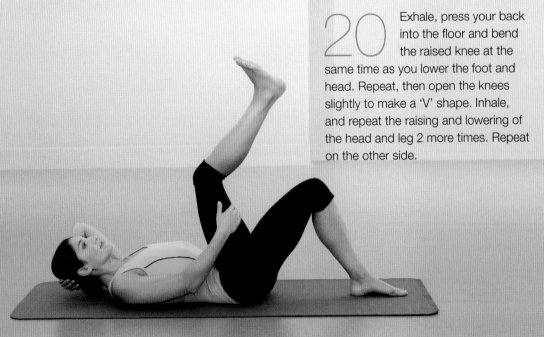

20 Exhale, press your back into the floor and bend the raised knee at the same time as you lower the foot and head. Repeat, then open the knees slightly to make a 'V' shape. Inhale, and repeat the raising and lowering of the head and leg 2 more times. Repeat on the other side.

>> ear tilt/chin tilt

21 **Ear tilt** Sit up tall, hips firmly planted on the floor, legs crossed comfortably in front. Anchor your shoulder blades. Tilt your ear to your shoulder, using your hand on the side of your head to gently deepen the stretch, while you reach down with your other hand to create a dynamic opposition. Hold and breathe.

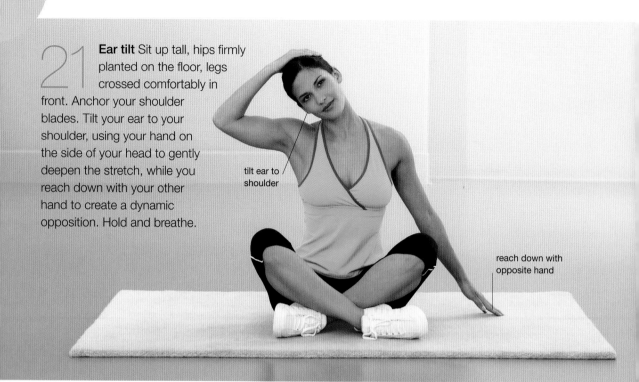

tilt ear to shoulder

reach down with opposite hand

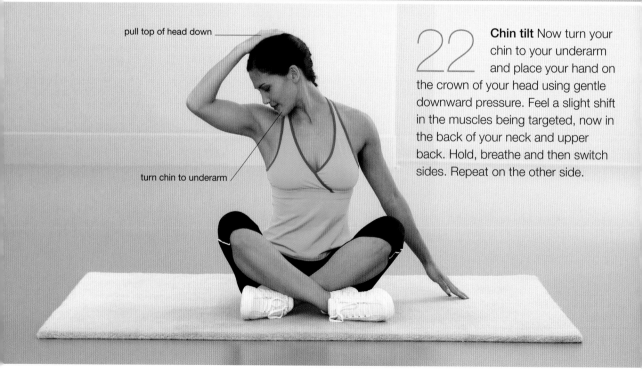

pull top of head down

turn chin to underarm

22 **Chin tilt** Now turn your chin to your underarm and place your hand on the crown of your head using gentle downward pressure. Feel a slight shift in the muscles being targeted, now in the back of your neck and upper back. Hold, breathe and then switch sides. Repeat on the other side.

>> **easy** seated

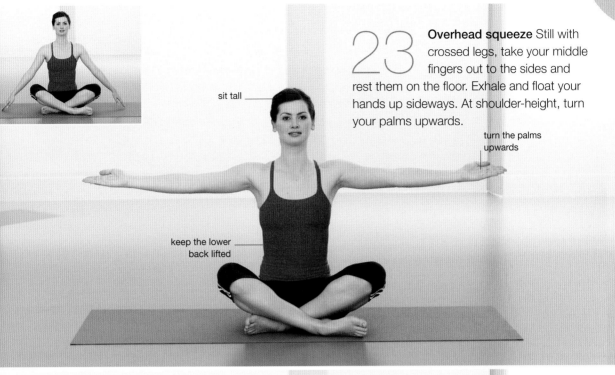

sit tall

turn the palms upwards

keep the lower back lifted

23 **Overhead squeeze** Still with crossed legs, take your middle fingers out to the sides and rest them on the floor. Exhale and float your hands up sideways. At shoulder-height, turn your palms upwards.

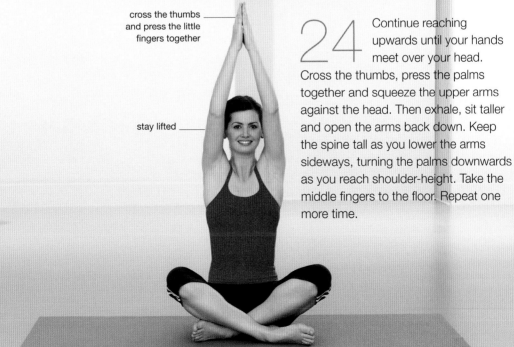

cross the thumbs and press the little fingers together

stay lifted

24 Continue reaching upwards until your hands meet over your head. Cross the thumbs, press the palms together and squeeze the upper arms against the head. Then exhale, sit taller and open the arms back down. Keep the spine tall as you lower the arms sideways, turning the palms downwards as you reach shoulder-height. Take the middle fingers to the floor. Repeat one more time.

>> side bends

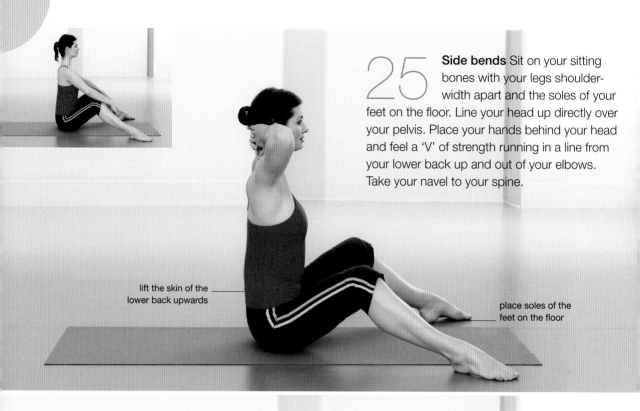

25 **Side bends** Sit on your sitting bones with your legs shoulder-width apart and the soles of your feet on the floor. Line your head up directly over your pelvis. Place your hands behind your head and feel a 'V' of strength running in a line from your lower back up and out of your elbows. Take your navel to your spine.

lift the skin of the lower back upwards

place soles of the feet on the floor

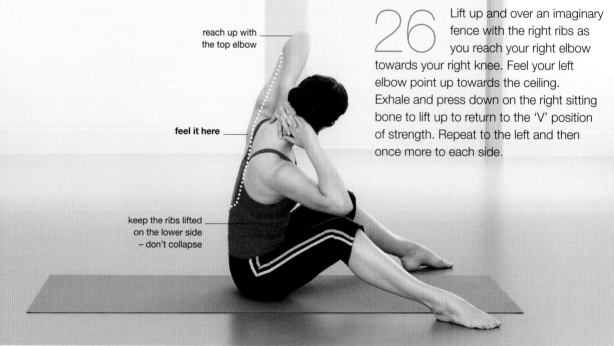

reach up with the top elbow

feel it here

keep the ribs lifted on the lower side – don't collapse

26 Lift up and over an imaginary fence with the right ribs as you reach your right elbow towards your right knee. Feel your left elbow point up towards the ceiling. Exhale and press down on the right sitting bone to lift up to return to the 'V' position of strength. Repeat to the left and then once more to each side.

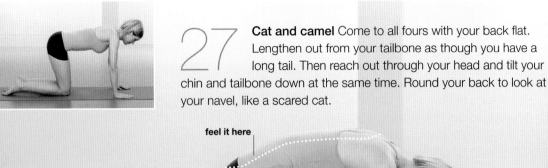

27 Cat and camel Come to all fours with your back flat. Lengthen out from your tailbone as though you have a long tail. Then reach out through your head and tilt your chin and tailbone down at the same time. Round your back to look at your navel, like a scared cat.

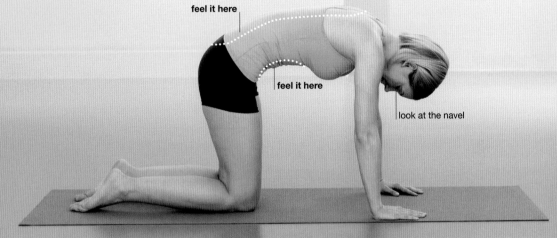

feel it here

feel it here

look at the navel

28 Exhale and lengthen backwards to flatten your back again, then look forwards and arch your back like a camel. Feel as if your tailbone could reach the top of your head. Repeat one more time. Return to the flat-back position and relax.

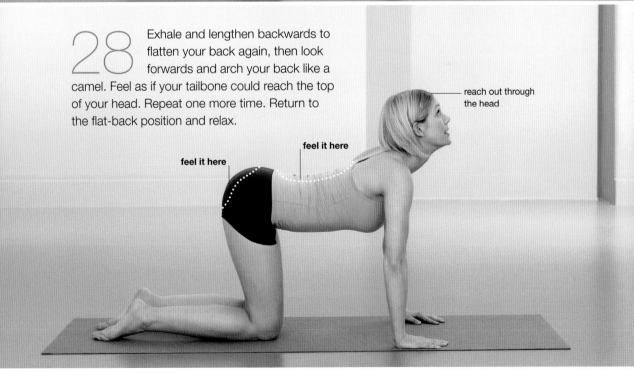

reach out through the head

feel it here

feel it here

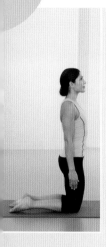

29 **Front body opener**
Kneel up, with your knees under your pelvis. Tuck your pelvis under and press your hips forwards. Reach your arms behind you and clasp your hands behind your back, without over-arching the back. Inhale, press your hips together, and squeeze your glutes. Lift your chest and stretch your hands behind you.

30 Exhale, relax your hands and come back to centre. Repeat another 2 times.

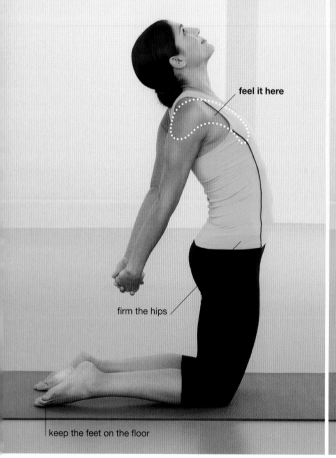

feel it here

firm the hips

keep the feet on the floor

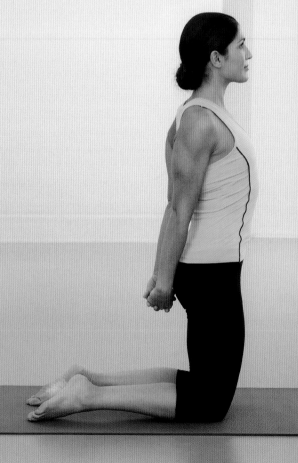

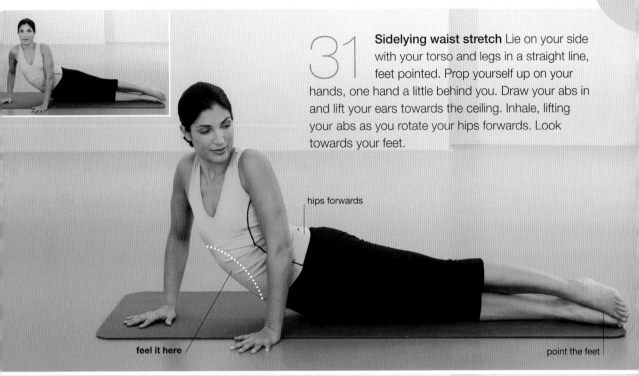

31 **Sidelying waist stretch** Lie on your side with your torso and legs in a straight line, feet pointed. Prop yourself up on your hands, one hand a little behind you. Draw your abs in and lift your ears towards the ceiling. Inhale, lifting your abs as you rotate your hips forwards. Look towards your feet.

hips forwards

feel it here

point the feet

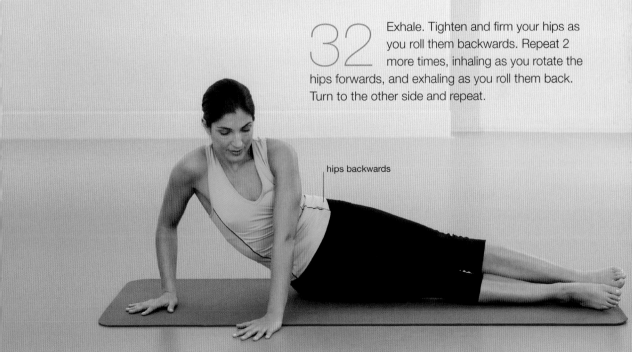

32 Exhale. Tighten and firm your hips as you roll them backwards. Repeat 2 more times, inhaling as you rotate the hips forwards, and exhaling as you roll them back. Turn to the other side and repeat.

hips backwards

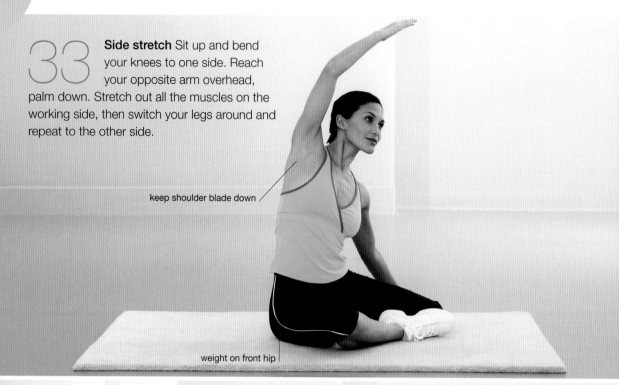

33 **Side stretch** Sit up and bend your knees to one side. Reach your opposite arm overhead, palm down. Stretch out all the muscles on the working side, then switch your legs around and repeat to the other side.

keep shoulder blade down

weight on front hip

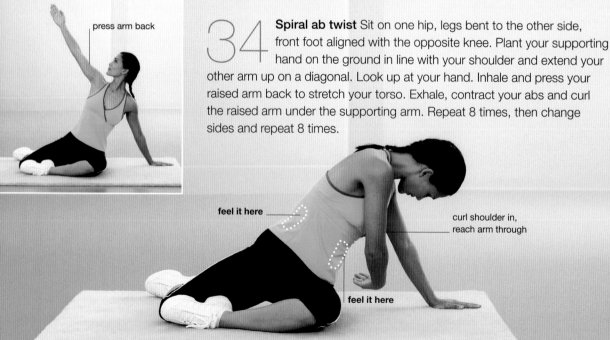

press arm back

34 **Spiral ab twist** Sit on one hip, legs bent to the other side, front foot aligned with the opposite knee. Plant your supporting hand on the ground in line with your shoulder and extend your other arm up on a diagonal. Look up at your hand. Inhale and press your raised arm back to stretch your torso. Exhale, contract your abs and curl the raised arm under the supporting arm. Repeat 8 times, then change sides and repeat 8 times.

feel it here

curl shoulder in, reach arm through

feel it here

35 **Cross-legged pose** Come to a cross-legged position. Inhale, exhale and relax forward as your sitting bones push down and back and your fingers inch forward on every exhalation. On each exhalation, let the torso hinge forward over your thighs to open the hips. If your knees hurt, push back and down with your buttocks and do not come so far forward. Come up to sitting, then cross your legs the other way and repeat.

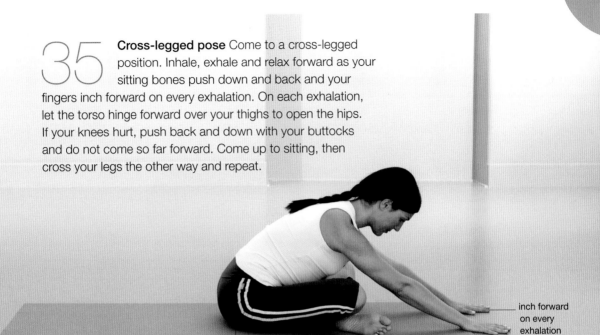

inch forward on every exhalation

root down and back

36 **Twist** Inhale and come up. Place your left hand on your right thigh and your right hand on the floor behind you. Turn your head and torso to the right. As you inhale, feel yourself getting taller. Exhale, twisting. Inhale and come back to the centre. Repeat on the other side.

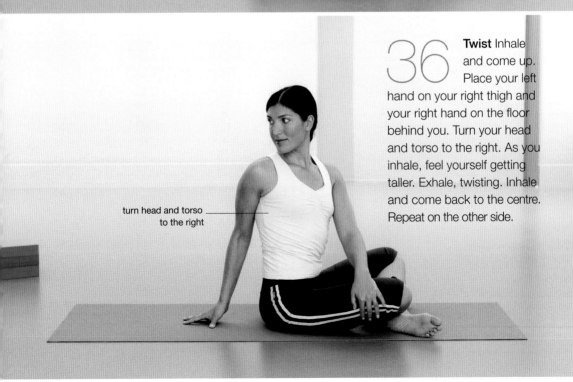

turn head and torso to the right

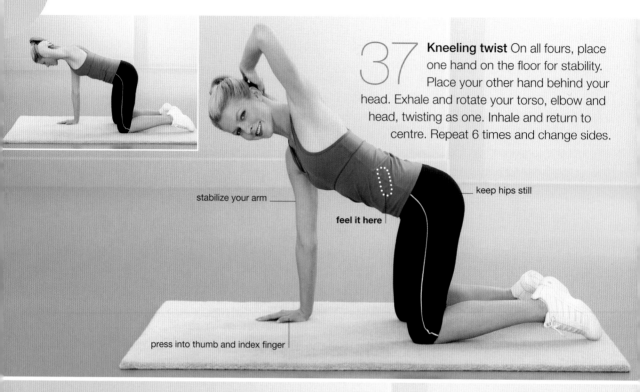

37 **Kneeling twist** On all fours, place one hand on the floor for stability. Place your other hand behind your head. Exhale and rotate your torso, elbow and head, twisting as one. Inhale and return to centre. Repeat 6 times and change sides.

stabilize your arm _____

keep hips still

feel it here

press into thumb and index finger

38 **Thread the needle** This is a Spinal twist from the knees. Starting on all fours, 'thread' one arm under your body to the opposite side, palm up. Come to rest on your shoulder and the side of your head. Breathe into the stretch, feeling the elongation all along your side. Then change sides and thread the needle the other way.

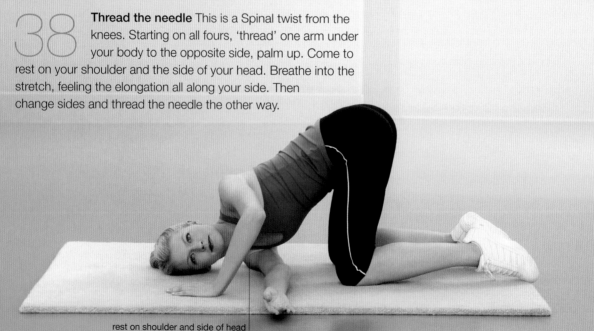

rest on shoulder and side of head

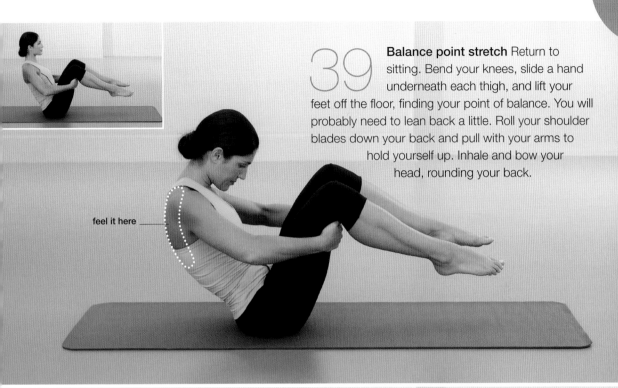

39 **Balance point stretch** Return to sitting. Bend your knees, slide a hand underneath each thigh, and lift your feet off the floor, finding your point of balance. You will probably need to lean back a little. Roll your shoulder blades down your back and pull with your arms to hold yourself up. Inhale and bow your head, rounding your back.

feel it here

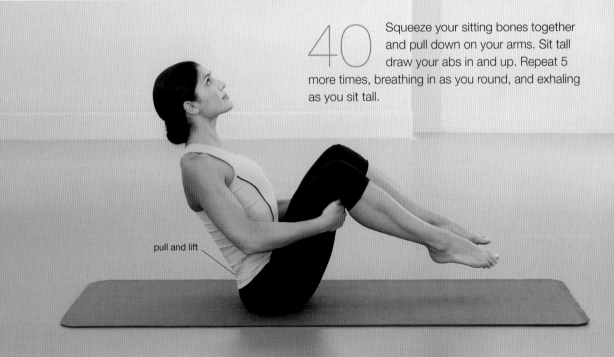

40 Squeeze your sitting bones together and pull down on your arms. Sit tall draw your abs in and up. Repeat 5 more times, breathing in as you round, and exhaling as you sit tall.

pull and lift

>> spine twist

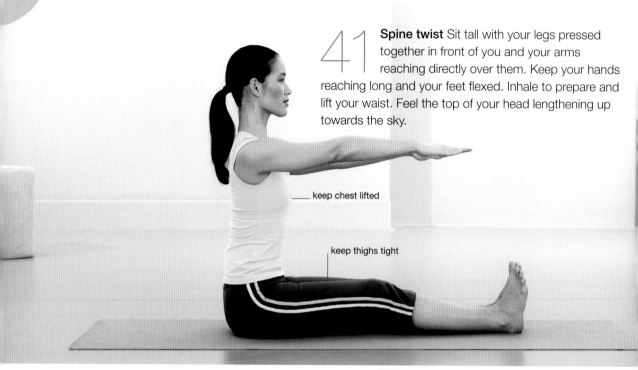

41 **Spine twist** Sit tall with your legs pressed together in front of you and your arms reaching directly over them. Keep your hands reaching long and your feet flexed. Inhale to prepare and lift your waist. Feel the top of your head lengthening up towards the sky.

keep chest lifted

keep thighs tight

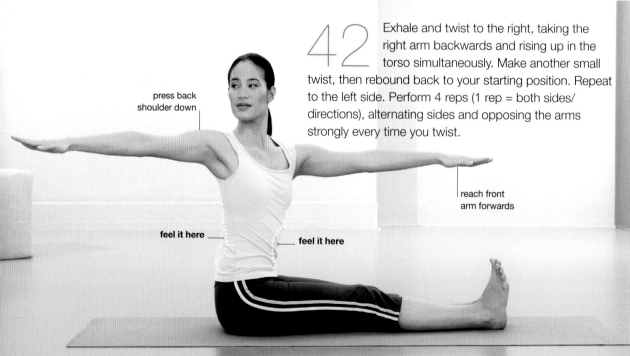

42 Exhale and twist to the right, taking the right arm backwards and rising up in the torso simultaneously. Make another small twist, then rebound back to your starting position. Repeat to the left side. Perform 4 reps (1 rep = both sides/ directions), alternating sides and opposing the arms strongly every time you twist.

press back shoulder down

reach front arm forwards

feel it here

feel it here

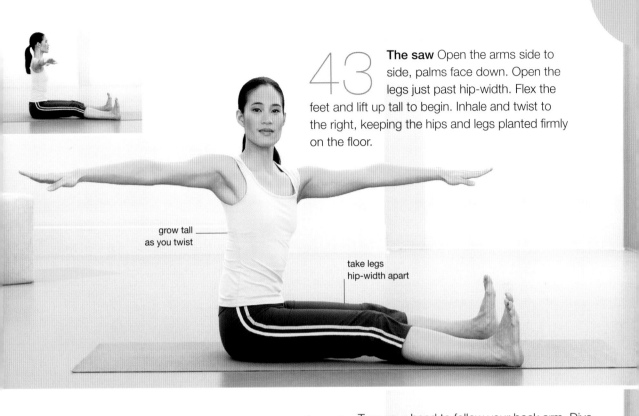

43 **The saw** Open the arms side to side, palms face down. Open the legs just past hip-width. Flex the feet and lift up tall to begin. Inhale and twist to the right, keeping the hips and legs planted firmly on the floor.

grow tall
as you twist

take legs
hip-width apart

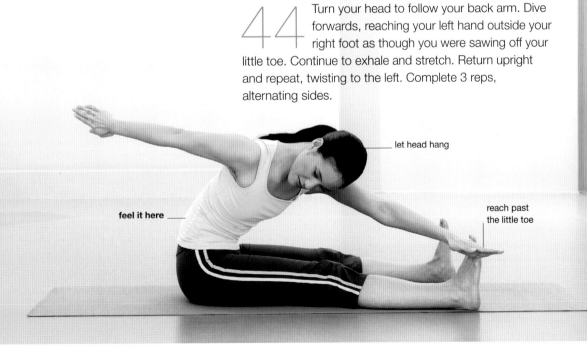

44 Turn your head to follow your back arm. Dive forwards, reaching your left hand outside your right foot as though you were sawing off your little toe. Continue to exhale and stretch. Return upright and repeat, twisting to the left. Complete 3 reps, alternating sides.

let head hang

feel it here

reach past
the little toe

easy seated >>

>> 'C' exercise

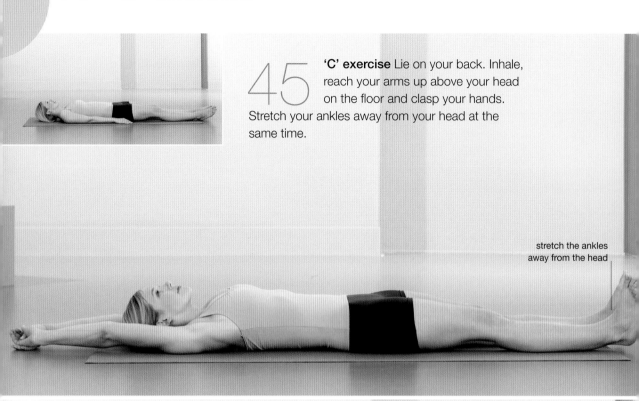

45 **'C' exercise** Lie on your back. Inhale, reach your arms up above your head on the floor and clasp your hands. Stretch your ankles away from your head at the same time.

stretch the ankles away from the head

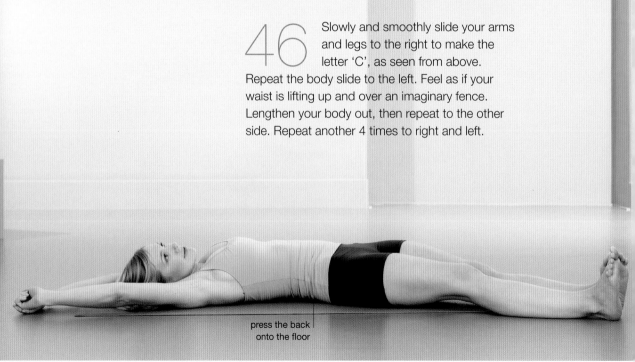

46 Slowly and smoothly slide your arms and legs to the right to make the letter 'C', as seen from above. Repeat the body slide to the left. Feel as if your waist is lifting up and over an imaginary fence. Lengthen your body out, then repeat to the other side. Repeat another 4 times to right and left.

press the back onto the floor

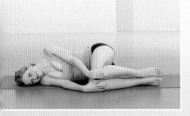

47 **Baby rolls** Lie on your right side with your legs bent up. Hold your hands on top of your knees. Roll onto your back, feeling as much of your back as possible resting against the floor.

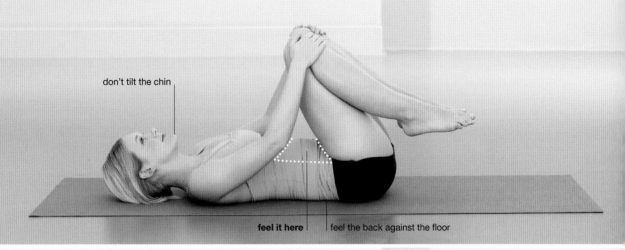

don't tilt the chin

feel it here | feel the back against the floor

48 Then roll over onto your left side, letting your focus and head linger to the right. Think: 'leg, leg', then the head rolls last. Repeat, starting on your left side, then rolling onto your back and lingering the focus to the left. Continue gently rolling from side to side 3 more times.

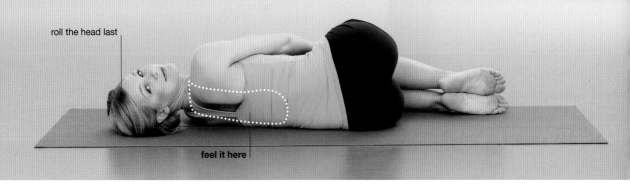

roll the head last

feel it here

>> arm fans

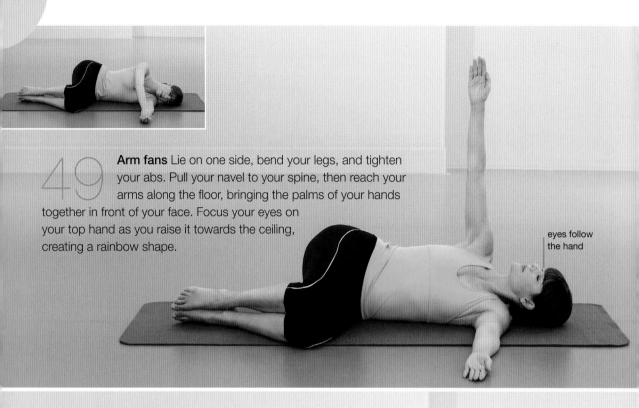

49 **Arm fans** Lie on one side, bend your legs, and tighten your abs. Pull your navel to your spine, then reach your arms along the floor, bringing the palms of your hands together in front of your face. Focus your eyes on your top hand as you raise it towards the ceiling, creating a rainbow shape.

eyes follow the hand

50 Continue moving the arm and reach behind you to the floor, allowing your shoulders and torso to rotate with the arm. Try not to move your knees. Exhale, then reach up with the hand as you reverse, 'painting the ceiling' with your fingertips until your hands are together again. Repeat 2 more times, inhaling as you open the arm, exhaling as you bring the palms together again. Roll over to the other side and repeat.

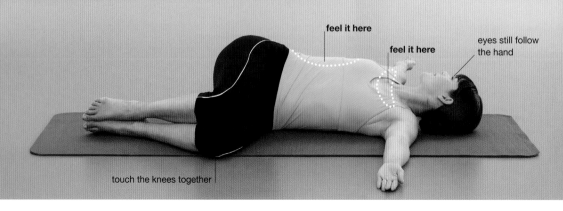

feel it here

feel it here

eyes still follow the hand

touch the knees together

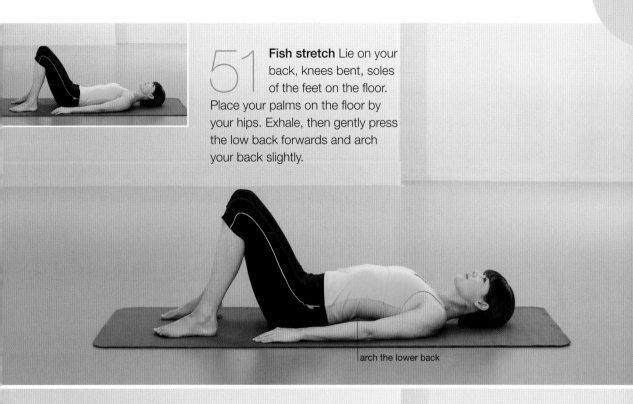

51 **Fish stretch** Lie on your back, knees bent, soles of the feet on the floor. Place your palms on the floor by your hips. Exhale, then gently press the low back forwards and arch your back slightly.

arch the lower back

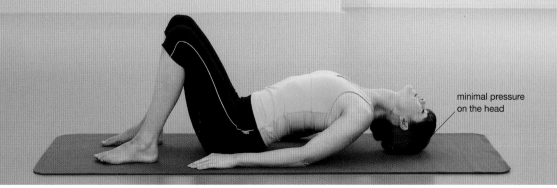

52 Roll your shoulder blades back and down, then press down on your forearms, and arch your back more to come up onto the top of your head. Put as little pressure on the head as possible. Stay for 1 long breath cycle. Relax, then repeat.

minimal pressure on the head

>> modified cobra

53 **Modified cobra** Go onto your stomach and firm and tighten your hips, pressing your thighs into the floor. Scoop your abs in, pulling your navel towards your spine. Reach your hands out onto the floor in front of you.

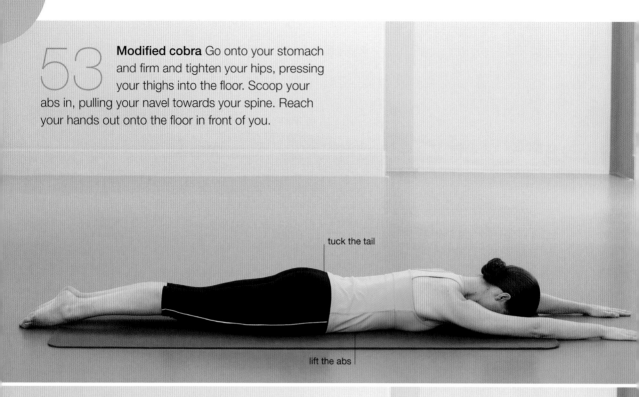

tuck the tail

lift the abs

54 Inhale as you drag your hands along the floor towards your shoulders, keeping the abs tight and lifting your front body so your ribs come off the floor. Exhale, slide the arms out in front of you, and take your face back to the floor. Repeat, then relax and breathe normally.

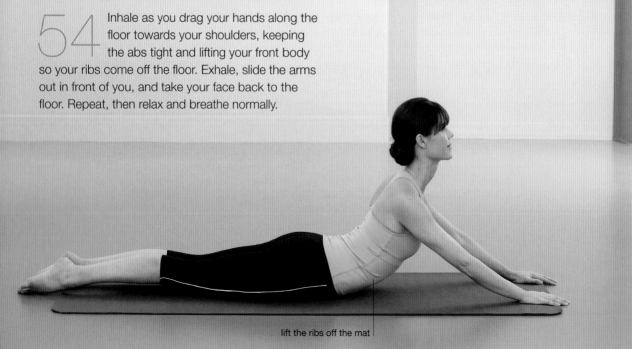

lift the ribs off the mat

>> **medium** prone

>> cobbler stretch

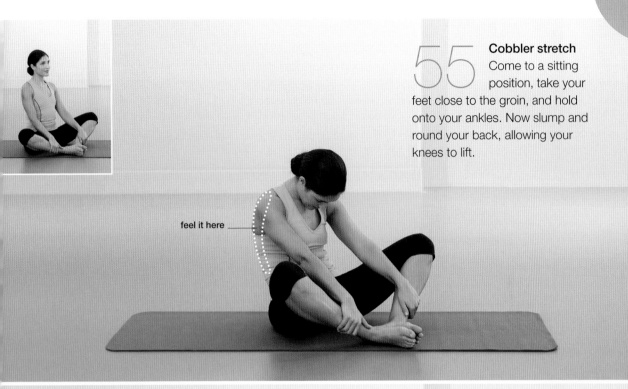

55 **Cobbler stretch**
Come to a sitting position, take your feet close to the groin, and hold onto your ankles. Now slump and round your back, allowing your knees to lift.

feel it here

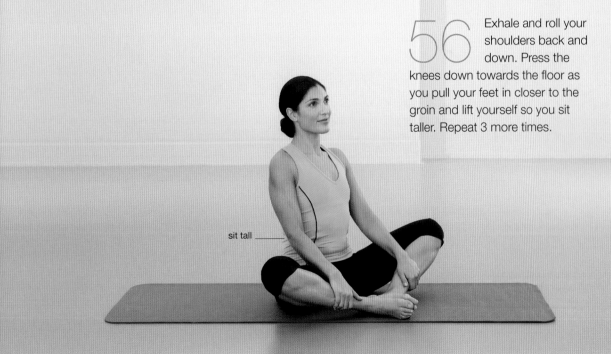

56 Exhale and roll your shoulders back and down. Press the knees down towards the floor as you pull your feet in closer to the groin and lift yourself so you sit taller. Repeat 3 more times.

sit tall

>> inverse frog

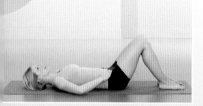

57 **Inverse frog** Lie on your back with bent knees. Compress your whole back against the floor and place your hands on your hips for feedback. Keep your back pressed firmly against the floor as you gently open both knees sideways towards the floor, like a frog. Let the soles of your feet come together.

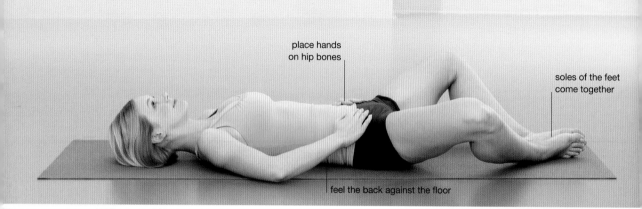

place hands on hip bones

soles of the feet come together

feel the back against the floor

58 Exhale and deepen the abdominal compression as you bring the knees together again. Repeat the frog-like opening and closing 3 more times. Relax.

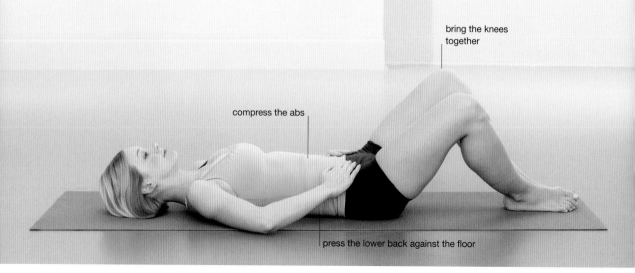

bring the knees together

compress the abs

press the lower back against the floor

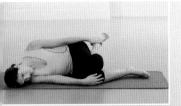

59 **Quad stretch** Lie on your side and bend both knees up towards your chest. Hold onto your bottom knee. Inhale, hold onto your top ankle and pull your top knee gently towards your chest.

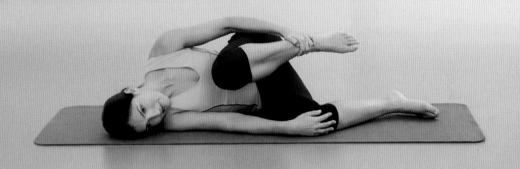

60 Exhale, then smoothly pull your top knee back. Do not let the bottom knee be pulled backwards by the top leg. Stay, then pull backwards a little more on the top knee. Repeat. Release your ankle and go onto your back, then return to your side and straighten your legs. Repeat, lying on the other side.

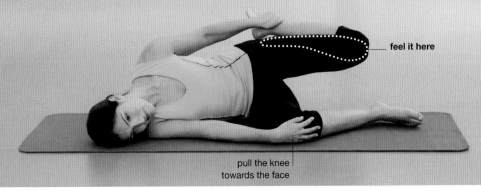

feel it here

pull the knee towards the face

>> thigh stretch

61 **Thigh stretch** Pick up your weights and come onto your knees, holding the weights with your arms extended directly in front of you just below shoulder-height. Face your palms down and tighten your abs to begin. Inhale to prepare.

62 Allow your chin to dip down slightly then hinge back, stretching the fronts of your thighs but not arching your spine. At your lowest point, tighten your buttocks and bring your body back up to start again. Perform a total of 4 times, exhaling each time you rise back up. Put the weights down.

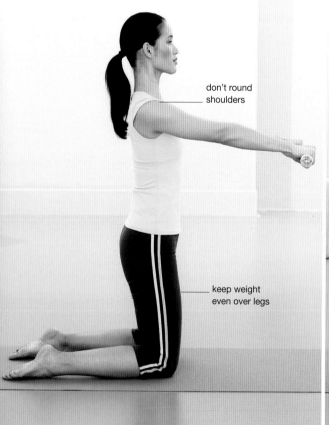

don't round shoulders

keep weight even over legs

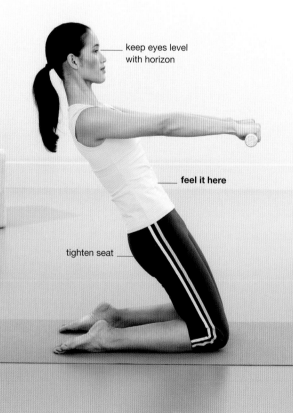

keep eyes level with horizon

feel it here

tighten seat

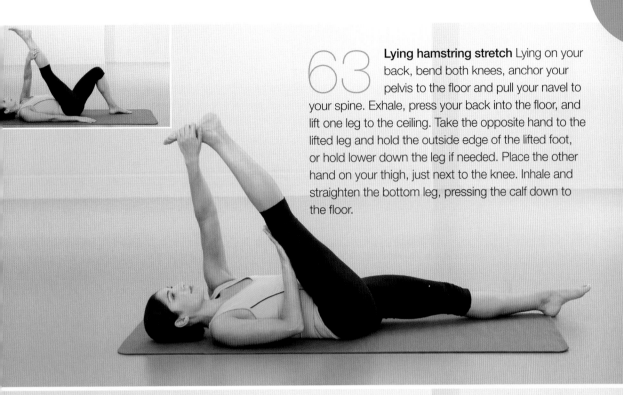

63 **Lying hamstring stretch** Lying on your back, bend both knees, anchor your pelvis to the floor and pull your navel to your spine. Exhale, press your back into the floor, and lift one leg to the ceiling. Take the opposite hand to the lifted leg and hold the outside edge of the lifted foot, or hold lower down the leg if needed. Place the other hand on your thigh, just next to the knee. Inhale and straighten the bottom leg, pressing the calf down to the floor.

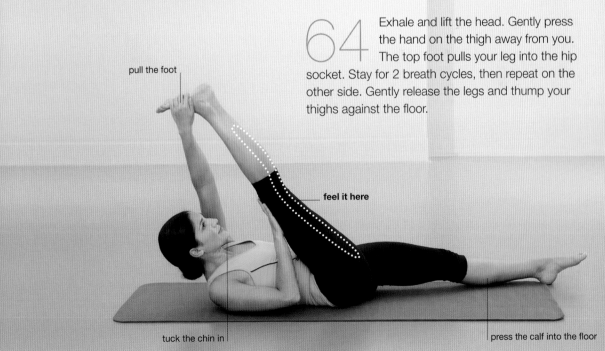

64 Exhale and lift the head. Gently press the hand on the thigh away from you. The top foot pulls your leg into the hip socket. Stay for 2 breath cycles, then repeat on the other side. Gently release the legs and thump your thighs against the floor.

pull the foot

feel it here

tuck the chin in

press the calf into the floor

>> figure 4 stretch

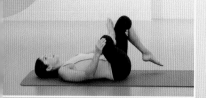

65 **Figure 4 stretch** Lying on your back, bend your knees and place one ankle on the other thigh. Place one hand underneath that thigh and the palm of the other hand on the knee of the crossed leg. Pull your abs tight to stabilize the spine. Inhale and pull the hand behind the thigh towards your chest.

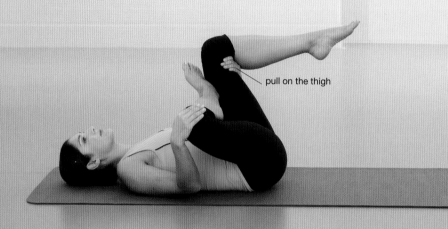

pull on the thigh

66 Exhale and press the hand against the knee, away from your face, keeping the bent leg parallel to the floor. If the knee hurts, come out of the position, or loosen the posture. Repeat. Release both legs, thump your thighs, and breathe normally. Repeat on the other side.

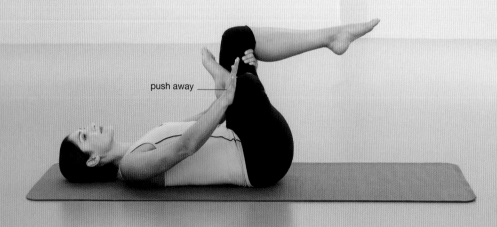

push away

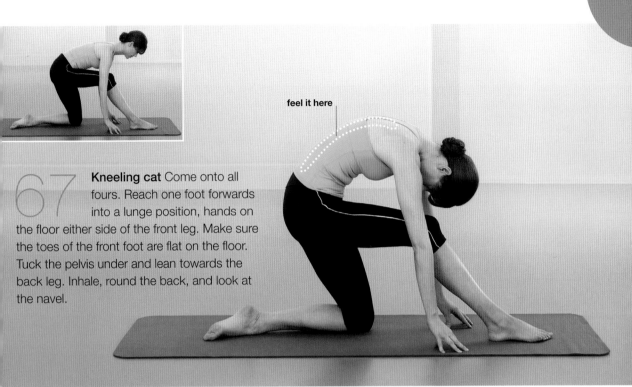

feel it here

67 **Kneeling cat** Come onto all fours. Reach one foot forwards into a lunge position, hands on the floor either side of the front leg. Make sure the toes of the front foot are flat on the floor. Tuck the pelvis under and lean towards the back leg. Inhale, round the back, and look at the navel.

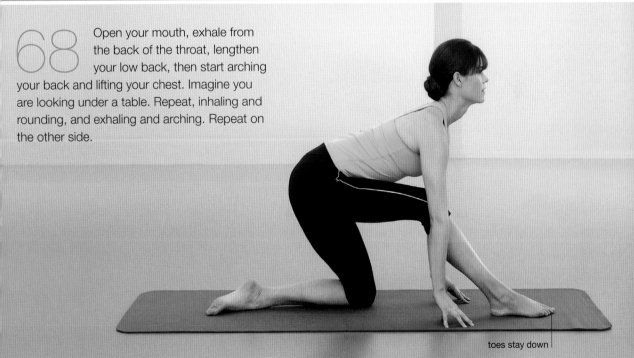

68 Open your mouth, exhale from the back of the throat, lengthen your low back, then start arching your back and lifting your chest. Imagine you are looking under a table. Repeat, inhaling and rounding, and exhaling and arching. Repeat on the other side.

toes stay down

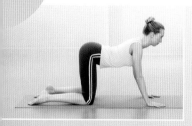

69 **Child's pose** Come to all fours, inhale and look ahead. Keep your shoulders away from your ears and your tailbone back. Exhale, rounding your back and looking towards your navel as you stretch your buttocks down towards your heels, with your head resting on the floor. Your hands are on the floor in front of you. At first, your head may not touch the floor and your buttocks may not reach your heels. If your knees feel very stiff, place a blanket behind the knees. If your ankles hurt, place a rolled towel under them.

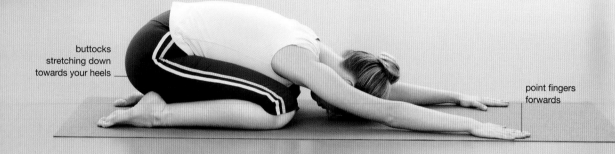

buttocks stretching down towards your heels

point fingers forwards

easier option

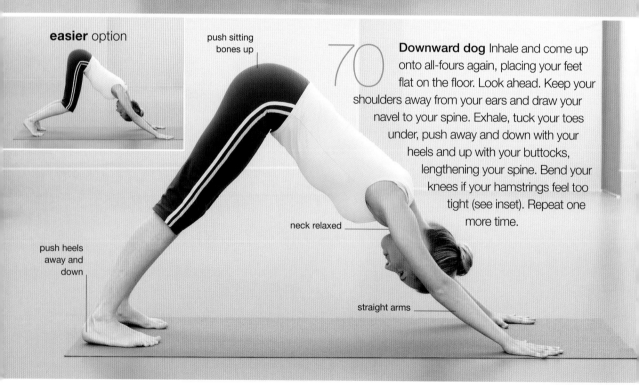

push sitting bones up

70 **Downward dog** Inhale and come up onto all-fours again, placing your feet flat on the floor. Look ahead. Keep your shoulders away from your ears and draw your navel to your spine. Exhale, tuck your toes under, push away and down with your heels and up with your buttocks, lengthening your spine. Bend your knees if your hamstrings feel too tight (see inset). Repeat one more time.

neck relaxed

push heels away and down

straight arms

71 **Forward bend** From step 70, gently walk your feet and hands towards each other, keeping your feet parallel and hip-width apart. If your back feels stiff, stop here, with your legs bent (see inset). Otherwise, lift your kneecaps and suck the front of your thighs up and back to straighten your legs.

72 **Mountain pose** Inhale and sweep your arms out to the side and up over your head as you come up to standing. Keep your legs straight and stretch all along the outside of your body to your fingertips.

arms reaching up

easier option

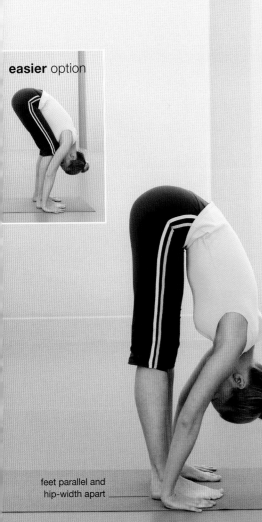

feet parallel and hip-width apart

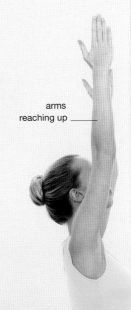

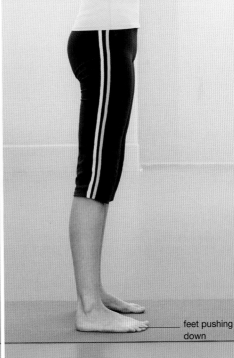

feet pushing down

>> pull-the-thread lunge

73 **Pull-the-thread lunge** Go onto all
fours, take one leg in front and lean
into it, palms either side of the front
foot. Line up the bent-leg knee and toes straight
ahead in front of the hip. Press the foot into the
floor. Extend the other leg straight behind you
and tuck the pelvis under strongly.

tuck the tail under _____

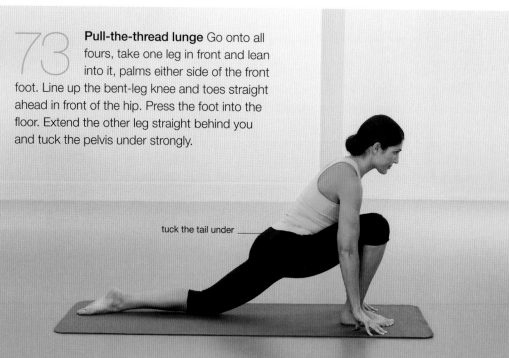

74 Pull an imaginary thread up to the
ceiling with the hand on the side
of the extended leg. Look up at
the hand and press down into the floor with the
other hand. Stay for 2 breath cycles. Take the
hand down to the floor, then repeat with the
other leg in front.

_____ look at the 'thread'

tighten the waist _____

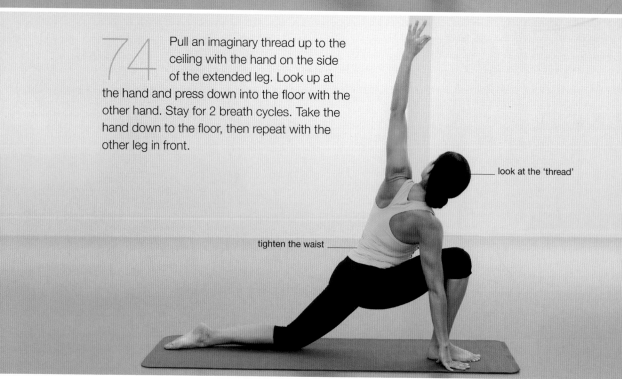

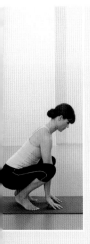

75 **Flat-back squat** Come into a squatting position. Let your knees open and go onto the balls of your feet. Lean on your hands, then inhale as you lift diagonally up and out with your chest, keeping your back flat and extended. Imagine you are looking under a table.

76 Exhale slowly as you lift your hips upwards, taking the heels as high as you can. Straighten your knees and tuck your chin into your legs. Keep holding your abs tight. Stay and breathe, then repeat, intensifying the stretch at the end. Lower and relax. Repeat, then lower.

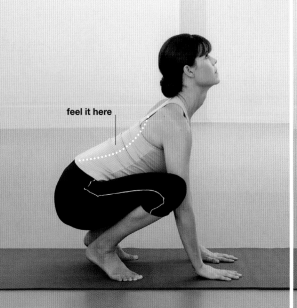

feel it here

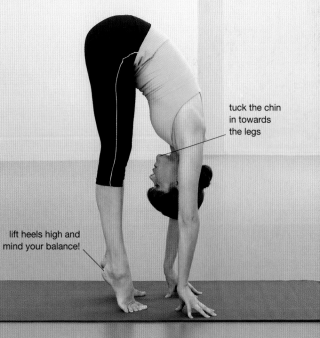

tuck the chin in towards the legs

lift heels high and mind your balance!

77 **The horse** Take your feet wide apart with your toes turned out 45°. Bend your knees so that they are in line with your feet and bring your hands to the front of your chest in prayer position. Hold for 2 breath cycles.

78 **Triangle** Inhale and straighten your legs. Stretch your arms out straight at shoulder-height. Turn your right foot out and your left foot in. Exhale and reach to the right, bringing your right hand to rest on your right shin and your left arm straight up. Inhale and look down at your front big toe. Exhale and look ahead. Take a couple of breaths then come up. Repeat on the left side.

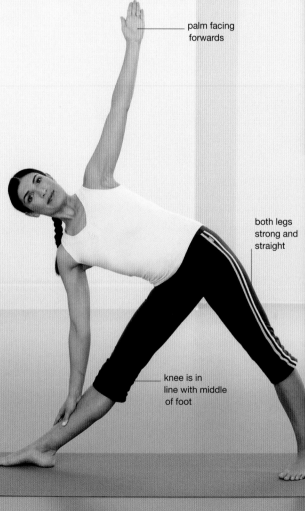

palm facing forwards

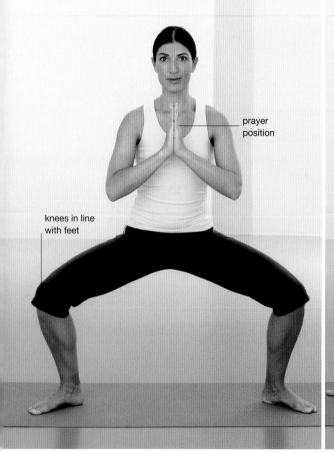

prayer position

both legs strong and straight

knees in line with feet

knee is in line with middle of foot

>> warrior 2/side-angle stretch

79 **Warrior 2** With feet apart, turn your right foot out and your left foot in. Exhale and bend your right knee directly over your ankle. Rotate both your knees away from each other. Keep strong and straight on your left leg all the way to the outside of your foot. Inhale and stretch your arms out, looking out towards your right index finger. Take a couple of breaths.

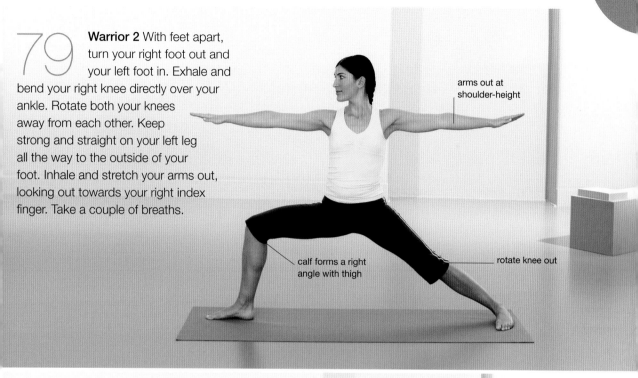

arms out at shoulder-height

calf forms a right angle with thigh

rotate knee out

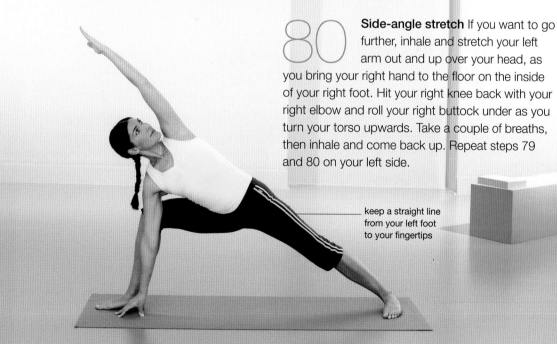

80 **Side-angle stretch** If you want to go further, inhale and stretch your left arm out and up over your head, as you bring your right hand to the floor on the inside of your right foot. Hit your right knee back with your right elbow and roll your right buttock under as you turn your torso upwards. Take a couple of breaths, then inhale and come back up. Repeat steps 79 and 80 on your left side.

keep a straight line from your left foot to your fingertips

>> oppositional lifts

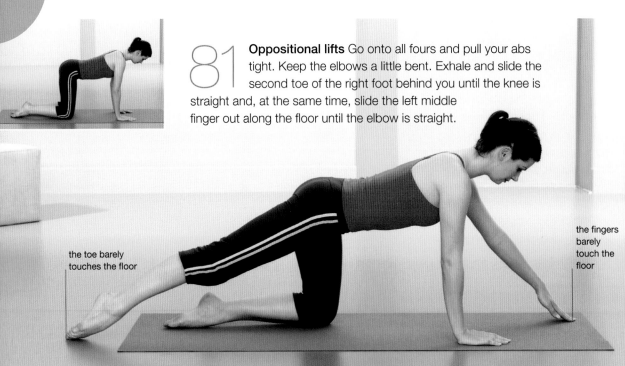

81 **Oppositional lifts** Go onto all fours and pull your abs tight. Keep the elbows a little bent. Exhale and slide the second toe of the right foot behind you until the knee is straight and, at the same time, slide the left middle finger out along the floor until the elbow is straight.

the toe barely touches the floor

the fingers barely touch the floor

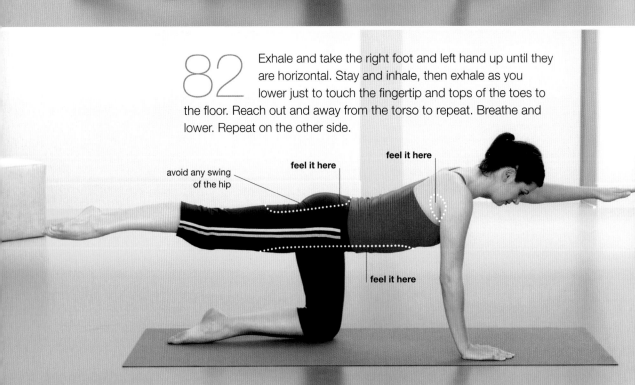

82 Exhale and take the right foot and left hand up until they are horizontal. Stay and inhale, then exhale as you lower just to touch the fingertip and tops of the toes to the floor. Reach out and away from the torso to repeat. Breathe and lower. Repeat on the other side.

avoid any swing of the hip

feel it here

feel it here

feel it here

83 **Advancing frogs** Come onto all fours, open your knees, reach your arms forwards, and squat back, bringing your hips close to your heels. Support your back by lifting the abs. Stay for 2 breath cycles.

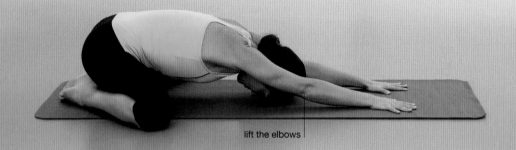

lift the elbows

84 Move your torso and arms forwards and come up onto your forearms. Actively press the inner edges of your heels into the floor. Your heels will come apart. Lift your abs in and up to avoid slumping in the low back. Stay for 2 breath cycles.

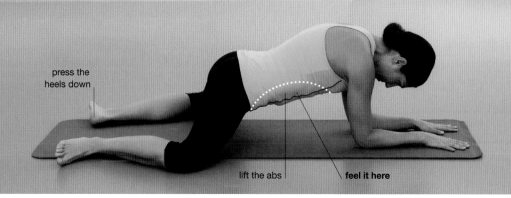

press the
heels down

lift the abs

feel it here

>> lunge opener

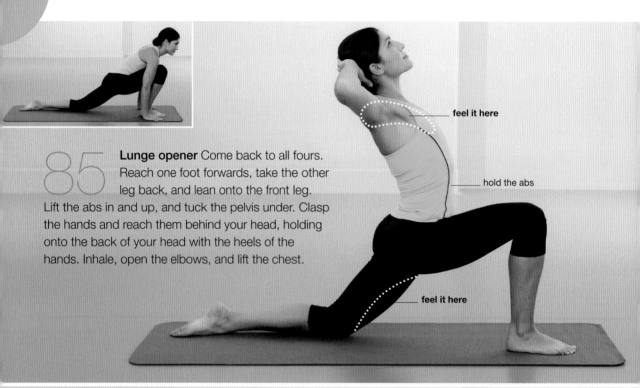

feel it here

hold the abs

85 **Lunge opener** Come back to all fours. Reach one foot forwards, take the other leg back, and lean onto the front leg. Lift the abs in and up, and tuck the pelvis under. Clasp the hands and reach them behind your head, holding onto the back of your head with the heels of the hands. Inhale, open the elbows, and lift the chest.

feel it here

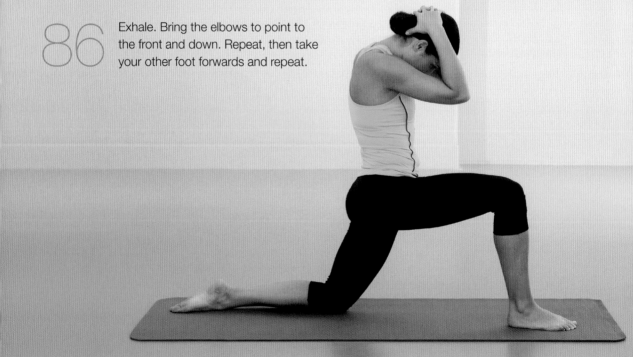

86 Exhale. Bring the elbows to point to the front and down. Repeat, then take your other foot forwards and repeat.

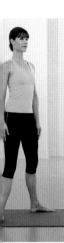

87 **Wide squat twist**
Come to a standing position with your feet wider than hip-width apart and your toes facing outwards. Lift your pelvic floor, inhale and lower your hips. Bring your hands to the thighs, take some of your weight into them, and check that your toes are in line with your knees.

88 Inhale, press backwards on one hand on the inside of the knee, twisting that shoulder down. Look up and out in the opposite direction. Stay for 2 breath cycles, then exhale and bring the shoulders back to centre. Come up, shake your legs a little, and repeat on the other side.

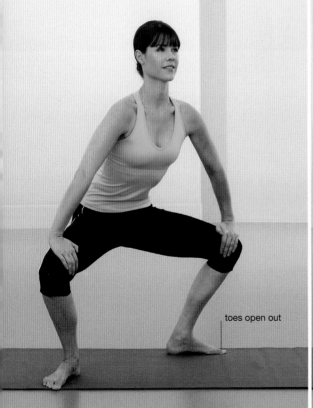

toes open out

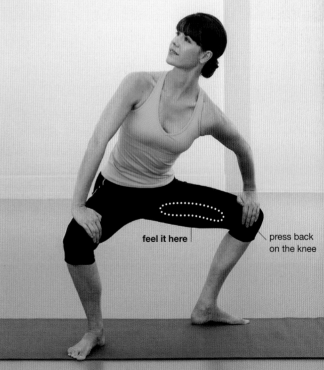

feel it here

press back on the knee

>> fouetté stretch

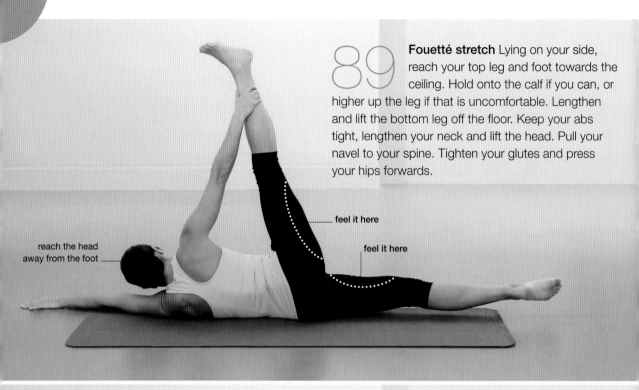

89 **Fouetté stretch** Lying on your side, reach your top leg and foot towards the ceiling. Hold onto the calf if you can, or higher up the leg if that is uncomfortable. Lengthen and lift the bottom leg off the floor. Keep your abs tight, lengthen your neck and lift the head. Pull your navel to your spine. Tighten your glutes and press your hips forwards.

feel it here

feel it here

reach the head away from the foot

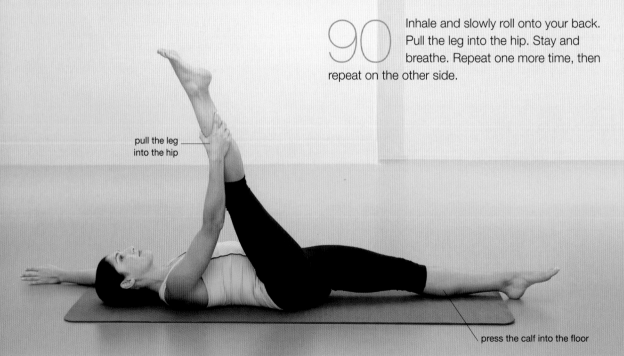

90 Inhale and slowly roll onto your back. Pull the leg into the hip. Stay and breathe. Repeat one more time, then repeat on the other side.

pull the leg into the hip

press the calf into the floor

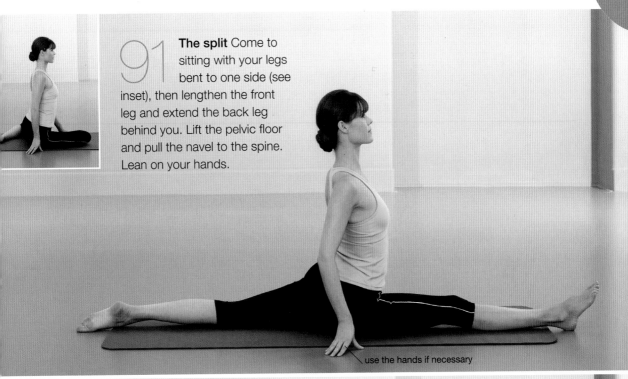

91 **The split** Come to sitting with your legs bent to one side (see inset), then lengthen the front leg and extend the back leg behind you. Lift the pelvic floor and pull the navel to the spine. Lean on your hands.

use the hands if necessary

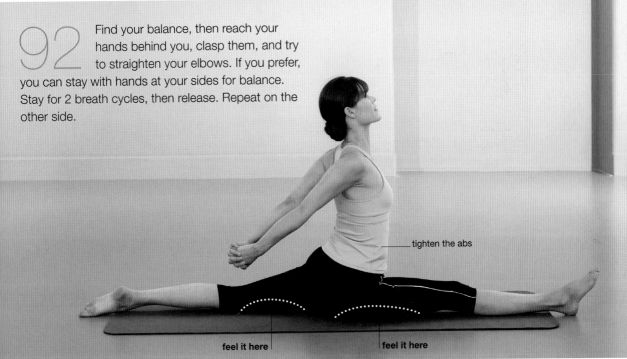

92 Find your balance, then reach your hands behind you, clasp them, and try to straighten your elbows. If you prefer, you can stay with hands at your sides for balance. Stay for 2 breath cycles, then release. Repeat on the other side.

tighten the abs

feel it here   feel it here

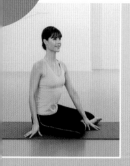

93 Pigeon arabesque
From a seated position, bend one leg back and the other forwards. Your legs should make a letter 'Z', with your front foot touching the back knee (see inset). Place your hands on the floor in front of you. Straighten the back leg behind you, with the knee pointing towards the floor.

tuck the tail under

balance on the thigh

94 Hold your position and reach the arm on the same side as the back leg out in front of you. Reach the arm on the bent-leg side out to the side. Stretch up through the head. Stay for 2 breath cycles, then switch legs and repeat.

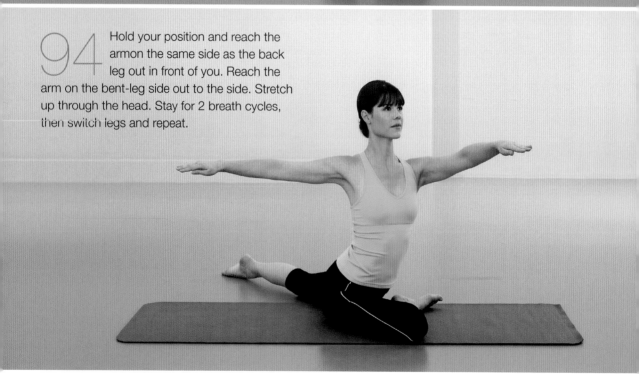

95 **Angel flight stretch** Lie on your stomach, face turned to one side. Scoop your abs in, drawing your navel to your spine. Press your tailbone down towards your heels. Inhale, then reach back and bend your knees to hold onto your ankles.

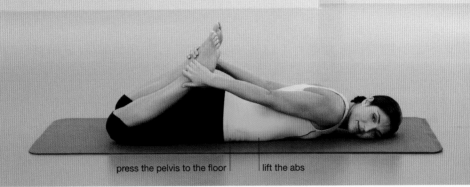

press the pelvis to the floor | lift the abs

96 Exhale, press your feet against your hands, and lift your chest and thighs off the floor to make a bow-like shape. Stay for 2 breath cycles, then release your hands and feet and relax for another 2 breath cycles, breathing deeply.

press the feet against the hands

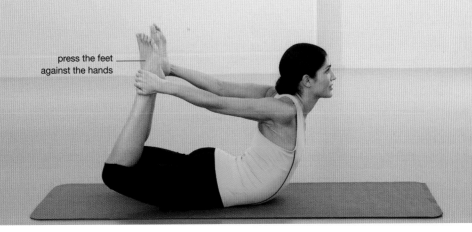

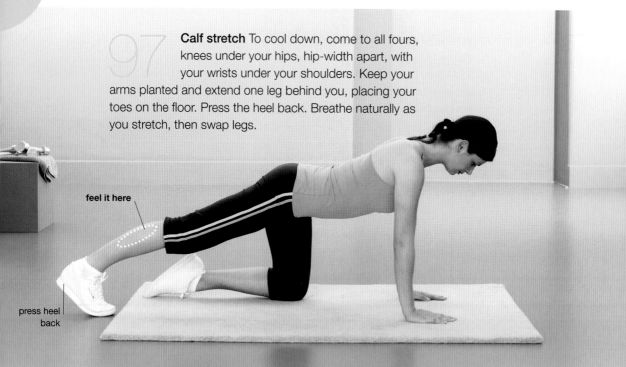

Calf stretch To cool down, come to all fours, knees under your hips, hip-width apart, with your wrists under your shoulders. Keep your arms planted and extend one leg behind you, placing your toes on the floor. Press the heel back. Breathe naturally as you stretch, then swap legs.

feel it here

press heel back

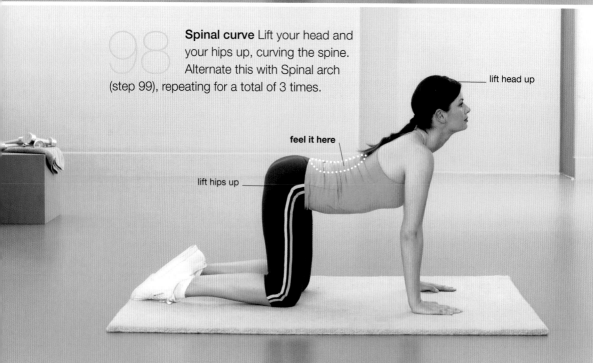

Spinal curve Lift your head and your hips up, curving the spine. Alternate this with Spinal arch (step 99), repeating for a total of 3 times.

lift head up

feel it here

lift hips up

Spinal arch Start from a kneeling positon, knees under hips, wrists under shoulders, your back neutral. Then arch your spine, rounding it up to the ceiling by tucking your hips under and dropping your head between your arms. Alternate this with Spinal curve (step 98), repeating for a total of 3 times.

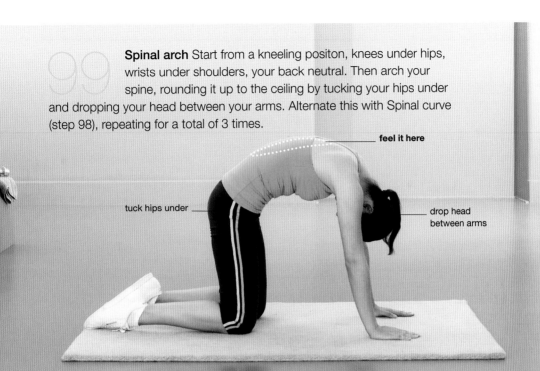

feel it here

tuck hips under

drop head between arms

Child's pose Sit back, reaching your hips towards your heels, at the same time rounding forward and extending your arms in front of you until your head rests on the floor. Keep your elbows off the floor to get the best stretch. Sink down into the position, holding for 3 deep breath cycles and sinking deeper into the position with each exhalation.

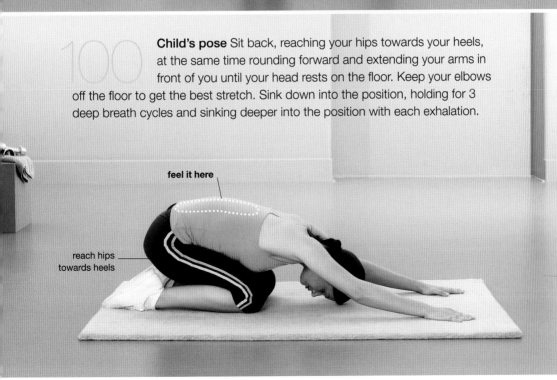

feel it here

reach hips towards heels

index

A

advancing frogs 53

angel flight stretch 59

arabesque, pigeon 58

arms: angel flight stretch 59

arm circles 13

arm fans 36

arm swing 12

butterfly stretch 16

'C' exercise 34

downward dog 46

elbow circles 15

mountain pose 47

overhead squeeze 23

pigeon arabesque 58

pull-the-thread lunge 48

shoulder circles 14

side-angle stretch 51

side bends 24

side stretch 28

spine twist 32

triangle 50

warrior 2 51

B

baby rocks 20

baby rolls 35

back: baby rolls 35

back stretch 17

balance point stretch 31

cat and camel 25

child's pose 46, 61

cobbler stretch 39

fish stretch 37

flat-back squat 49

hanging stretch 18

kneeling cat 45

modified cobra 38

pull-the-thread lunge 48

the saw 33

side bends 24

spinal arch 61

spinal curve 60

spine twist 32

thread the needle 30

balance point stretch 31

butterfly stretch 16

buttocks: baby rocks 20

cat and camel 25

oppositional lifts 52

C

'C' exercise 34

calf stretch 60

camel 25

cat, kneeling 45

cat and camel 25

chest: angel flight stretch 59

arm fans 36

back stretch 17

butterfly stretch 16

front body opener 26

lunge opener 54

child's pose 46, 61

chin tilt 22

cobbler stretch 39

cobra, modified 38

cooling-down 60–1

cross-legged pose 29

crunch with scoop 8

D

downward dog 46

E

ear tilt 22

elbow circles 15

F

fans, arm 36

figure 4 stretch 44

fish stretch 37

fitness, testing 8

flat-back squat 49

forward bend 47

fouetté stretch 56

frog, inverse 40

frogs, advancing 53

front body opener 26

H

half push-up 8

hamstrings: lying hamstring stretch 43

modifying exercises 10, 11

hanging stretch 18

hips: baby rocks 20

the horse 50

I

inverse frog 40

K

kneeling cat 45

kneeling twist 30

knees: knee pumps 21

painful 10, 11

L

legs: advancing frogs 53

'C' exercise 34

calf stretch 60

cross-legged pose 29

downward dog 46

figure 4 stretch 44

flat-back squat 49

forward bend 47

fouetté stretch 56

the horse 50

inverse frog 40

knee pumps 21

lunge opener 54

lying hamstring stretch 43

modifying exercises 10, 11

mountain pose 47

oppositional lifts 52

pigeon arabesque 58

quad stretch 41

side-angle stretch 51

the split 57

thigh stretch 42

triangle 50

warrior 2 51

wide squat twist 55

limbering up 12–19

lunges: lunge opener 54

    pull-the-thread lunge 48

lying hamstring stretch 43

M

modified cobra 38

modifying exercises 10–11

mountain pose 47

muscles, testing fitness 8

N

neck: chin tilt 22

    ear tilt 22

O

oppositional lifts 52

overhead squeeze 23

P

pain, modifying exercises 10, 11

PAR-Q questionnaire 9

pigeon arabesque 58

pull-the-thread lunge 48

push-up, half 8

Q

quad stretch 41

R

repetitions 8

rocking, baby rocks 20

rolls, baby 35

S

the saw 33

shoulders: front body opener 26

    shoulder circles 14

    shoulder ovals 19

side-angle stretch 51

side bends 24

side stretch 28

sidelying waist stretch 27

spinal arch 61

spinal curve 60

spine twist 32

spiral ab twist 28

the split 57

squats: flat-back squat 49

    wall squat 8

    wide squat twist 55

straps, modifying exercises 11

T

thighs: fouetté stretch 56

    the horse 50

    lunge opener 54

    lying hamstring stretch 43

    oppositional lifts 52

    pigeon arabesque 58

    quad stretch 41

    side-angle stretch 51

    the split 57

    thigh stretch 42

    wide squat twist 55

thread the needle 30

torso: advancing frogs 53

    angel flight stretch 59

    arm fans 36

    baby rolls 35

    back stretch 17

    cat and camel 25

    front body opener 26

    kneeling twist 30

    lunge opener 54

    oppositional lifts 52

    shoulder ovals 19

    side bends 24

    sidelying waist stretch 27

    spine twist 32

    spiral ab twist 28

    thigh stretch 42

twist 29

towels, modifying exercises 11

triangle 50

twists 29

    kneeling twist 30

    spine twist 32

    spiral ab twist 28

    wide squat twist 55

W

waist stretch, sidelying 27

wall squat 8

warming up 12–19

warrior 2 51

wide squat twist 55

acknowledgments

Publisher's acknowledgments

Dorling Kindersley would like to thank photographer Ruth Jenkinson and her assistants, Ann Burke, James McNaught, Carly Churchill and Vic Churchill: sweatyBetty for the loan of some of the exercise clothing; Viv Riley at Touch Studios; the models Jacqui Freeman, Carla Collins, Kerry Jay, Rhona Crewe, Sam Magee, Tara Lee, and Samantha Johannesson; Rachel Jones, Brigitta Smart, Roisin Donaghy and Victoria Barnes for the hair and makeup; YogaMatters for lending us the mat and other equipment. Anna Toombs and David Robinson of TR Balance for additional training support. A special thanks to Hilary Bird for the index. All images © Dorling Kindersley. For further information see **www.dkimages.com**

Original book acknowledgments:
Project Editors Helen Murray, Hilary Mandleberg
Project Art Editors Anne Fisher, Ruth Hope, Helen McTeer
Senior Editors Jennifer Latham, Jo Godfrey Wood
Senior Art Editors Peggy Sadler, Miranda Harvey, Susan Downing
Managing Editors Penny Warren, Dawn Henderson
Managing Art Editors Marianne Markham, Christine Keilty

about the authors

Joan Pagano, a Phi Beta Kappa, cum laude graduate of Connecticut College, is certified in health and fitness instruction by the American College of Sports Medicine (ACSM), whose credentials provide the very best measure of competence as a professional. She has worked as a personal fitness trainer on Manhatten's Upper East Side since 1988, providing professional guidance and support to people at all levels of fitness. Through her work, she has created hundreds of training programmes specially tailored for individuals, groups, fitness facilities, schools, hospitals, and corporations. Today, Joan manages her own staff of fitness specialists, who work together as Joan Pagano Fitness Group. For many years, she served as Director of the Personal Trainer Certification Program at Marymount Manhatten College, where she remains on the faculty as the instructor in fitness evaluation techniques. She is now a nationally recognized provider of education courses for fitness trainers through IDEA (an organization supporting fitness professionals worldwide). Joan is also recognized in the industry as an authority on the benefit of exercise for women's health issues such as pregnancy, the menopause, breast cancer, and osteoporosis.

Suzanne Martin is a doctor of physical therapy and a gold-certified Pilates expert. A former dancer, she is a Master trainer certified by the American Council on Exercise. She is also well known as an educational presenter within the world of Pilates, dance and physical therapy. Suzanne is the lead physical therapist for the Smuin Ballet in San Francisco and maintains a private practice, Total Body Development, in Alameda, California. For more information, check her website www.totalbodydevelopment.com

Efua Baker started her professional life as a dancer and fashion model. For the past 15 years she has been a personal trainer or "body sculptor" and her focus is always to ensure her clients look good and feel great; her unique and highly effective "body turnaround" techniques are much sought-after. Her workout style draws from many disciplines including dance, body-building, martial arts, yoga, and boxing.